Personal Safety Nets

Getting Ready for Life's Inevitable

Changes and Challenges

Dr. John W. Gibson

and

Judy Pigott

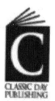

Classic Day Publishing

2925 Fairview Avenue East

Seattle, Washington 98102

206-860-4900

info@peanutbutterpublishing.com

Praise for Personal Safety Nets

How wonderful to bottle up the energy and wisdom of John and Judy. In their book, Personal Safety Nets, you'll find a clear and concise formula to use when you, your family, friends or associates need help in managing challenging issues of care. I've observed their work with families and have seen the benefit of clear communication and sharing the care. It's one fine book.

– Vanessa Carr, Director, www.CareAtHomeSeattle.com

This book presents an exquisite project—serious, rewarding, and offering a great opportunity for new learning. The two writers offer a wealth of thoughts, ideas, plans, opportunities, challenges and more on how we all could learn to support a care partner and his family in case of life changes.

The book is a wise, considerate, and extensive work based on hands-on experience and full of love and dedication to a cause of utmost worth for all sides involved.

In a world that seemingly grows colder and colder, this book encourages us all to come together and find our humanness anew. The care team offers such a beautiful opportunity, and here we find countless ideas presented in a most human way.

– Peter Kessler, lic.oec.HSG, Jona-Kempraten, Switzerland

John Gibson and Judy Pigott have written a powerful book with several important messages that have the potential to make aging and managing illness far more rewarding than our culture has yet allowed them to be. It's hard to explain to those who haven't had—and deeply fear—serious or life-threatening health challenges that the benefits can far outweigh the liabilities. Chief among the benefits is how being a care partner provides a great opportunity to depend on people who will grow profoundly from that experience, as we ourselves also are enriched from being able to count on support from others. This road map will help us let go of our isolation and unnecessary self-reliance.

– Denise Klein, Executive Director, Senior Services

Odds are that one day you will find yourself in the role of caregiver. This important book will help you to face the challenges of this role, and even more important, show you how to grow from the experience. It is all about having a personal safety net in place when such challenges come your way.

– Nancy J. Dapper, Executive Director, Western and Central
Washington Chapter of the Alzheimer's Association

In each of our lives there is a time when we need others in a way that we don't expect. Often challenging problems, such as caring for a spouse or family member, come when physical and economic difficulties make solutions seem impossible. Personal Safety Nets is a practical guide through the process of caring for self and others during difficult life experiences. It will help you gather resources around you in order to make your life and other lives successful, meaningful, and joyful. I highly recommend this book to family and friends of anyone going through a major health problem.

– Peter Grimm, MD, Director, Seattle Prostate Institute

This book strikes at the heart of both the challenges and joys of caring for a spouse or family who face illness, chronic disease, and end-of-life decision making. The authors are sensitive and address the uniqueness of each person's journey through the last chapter of one's life. A must read for families going through the maze and emotional roller coaster of eldercare.

– Mary Lynn Pannen, RN, CCM, President/CEO, Sound Options, Inc.

This book is a valuable tool for cancer patients and their caregivers.

– Susan Gordon, RN, Oncology, Fred Hutchinson Cancer Research Center

As I was helping John Gibson and Judy Pigott prepare this manuscript for publication, little did I know that they were actually preparing me to face the loss of my beloved grandmother, who died unexpectedly this spring. That's when I knew that John and Judy's collective wisdom and stories were far more than words on a page. As I was suddenly thrust into the role of griever and care team member all at once, with this book fresh in my mind, I almost felt as if John and Judy were standing by, comforting and coaching me. Becoming familiar with the stages of grief, recognizing boundaries, and identifying strong emotions were practical tools that I could use right away. I encourage readers to take time to read this book and discover that you can be well equipped to meet life's challenges—and stronger than you ever imagined.

– Karen Parkin, editor

As a family physician, I believe all my patients would benefit from having a personal safety net. Gibson and Pigott have done a great job of writing a "how-to" book on personal safety nets and on setting up care-sharing teams.

– Scott T. McIntyre, M.D., Seattle Primary Physicians, P.L.L.C.,
Seattle Family Medicine

In Personal Safety Nets, John Gibson and Judy Pigott provide a straightforward, flexible plan for navigating life-threatening and life-altering crises. It's a wonderfully practical, hopeful look at how forming supportive teams can help us in our darkest hours.

– Ann Marie Pomerinke, Chief Executive Officer, Great West
Division, Inc., American Cancer Society

Personal Safety Nets speaks to a truth I have both experienced and practiced. In my own personal life, in times of stress, I have children and friends upon whom I can call instantly; and they respond, always. I understand that I have been immeasurably blessed . . . and cannot imagine those times of ill health, sadness and stress without those dear wonderful souls.

As the former executive director of the Program for Early Parent Support (PEPS), I worked for twelve years developing and implementing parent support groups for families with children birth to three. The personal safety nets those groups formed were profound. Nothing is as scary as being a new parent. Nothing is as compelling as discovering mutual support and safety during that scary time.

Currently, I serve as CEO at Camp Fire USA Central Puget Sound Council. Again, I work with youth and families who form groups around a variety of programs; and from those groups, form personal safety nets that often begin when children are small and that last a lifetime.

I am convinced that support, through the context of safe and secure group networks, contributes mightily to our humanity and ability to deal with both life's joys and sorrows. Personal Safety Nets eloquently speaks to this phenomenon.

– Jane White Vulliet, CEO, Camp Fire USA Central Puget Sound Council (former ED, Program for Early Parent Support)

I am in the planning stages of building a care-team program for low-income single mothers and domestic violence survivors who often find themselves socially isolated at a time when they are most vulnerable. I was delighted to have Personal Safety Nets to fall into for practical advice and encouragement. The authors obviously have extensive experience with different kinds of care teams. They do not gloss over difficulties that may arise in teams or with partners, but rather show how to work through challenges realistically and with compassion for all concerned.

– Donna Pierce, Executive Director, Westside Baby

*To all the people who have been part
of our own personal safety nets and
have helped us learn how to create
and draw upon them.*

Whatever you do will not be enough,
but it matters enormously that you do it.
– Mahatma Gandhi

Table of Contents

Foreword

This is a much-needed book. Support networks don't just happen by themselves. These two experienced, compassionate experts have provided a realistic map and plan on how to help create and be part of a trusted, supportive network.

Why we all need such a network is becoming more important than ever. Health care insurance plans are being trimmed back or taken away from retirees; hospitals don't let patients occupy beds very long; and all government social and health-care services are being cut way back. Who can you count on? Your personal support network.

Psychology researchers have found, over and over, that resiliency, health, and long life are enhanced by having many good relationships and friendships. Loners, in contrast, don't hold up as well when struggling with long-lasting physical, emotional, or situational challenges.

Being part of a community of friendly people who enjoy many good times together has many benefits. If anyone is hit with a major personal difficulty, others are available to help in many ways. They may console, problem solve, bring food, take care of pets, provide transportation, wash dishes, fill out forms, rent a movie to watch together . . . the list goes on.

Enjoying good times together is an essential factor. Resiliency, recovery, and health are enhanced by many positive emotions. A good support group has many pleasant, happy people who laugh a lot, talk about many satisfactions in the work they do and in their lives, express appreciation, give hugs, delight in the accomplishments of others, and have a realistic optimistic attitude about handling challenges.

The wisdom offered to you by John and Judy is shown in their guidelines on how to receive help. When you face a serious difficulty, you may have to make a significant shift in your feelings about receiving help from others.

For example, a few years ago a friend of mine was seriously injured in an auto accident. She had fractured ribs, a fractured pelvis, and massive bruising. When she was recovered enough to be released from the hospital, she faced a dilemma. She had to remain in bed for many days while her bones mended, but she lived alone in a small house. She needed twenty-four-hour care in case any complications developed. She needed help with eating, going to the bathroom, turning the lights off and on, setting the thermostat, and so forth.

For her, the hardest part of her recovery was to accept an offer from two friends to go live in their home and let them care for her. She was an independent woman! She had always been generous in giving help to others. To accept help from others was more difficult for her than dealing with the pain of her broken body.

Now, when talking about the accident she says, "The biggest gift was learning to receive love. In the past I would never complain nor accept help from others. Now I do."

John and Judy are experienced guides who can lead you through the challenge of learning to ask for and receive help—if you are willing to accept their guidance. They speak from personal experience about what they have had to learn on their own.

John comes from a midwestern farming community and a large family of survivors. When he was fifteen years old, his mother had a massive stroke from which she did not recover. His older sister died in her thirties of cancer. John, his father, and his remaining sister have learned to rely on inner resources and an outer safety net to survive tragedy. He remembers a very difficult time when one of his cousins was killed in a flying accident. This was the second of three sons his uncle Bob had lost. John's father and another uncle felt Bob's pain very deeply because they had each also lost children who were in their twenties or thirties. After the funeral Bob said, "I don't know how I can go on." John's father replied, "Bob, we're survivors. And we have each other." The two brothers put their arms around Bob and held him as he sobbed in deep agony over his loss. In the months that followed, Bob recovered and the family healed from another tragic loss.

John served two years in the Army medical corps, counseling returning Vietnam veterans who had been traumatized by what they'd seen and experienced. In his professional career, he has focused on helping individuals and families find strength, adaptability, and community to draw upon during life's changes and challenges. His work with clients has given him many insights into how to create and sustain support networks.

Life has a way of making experts walk their talk. John personally knows what it's like to rely on a safety net. He developed a form of non-Hodgkin's lymphoma several years ago. He refers to it as "currently incurable" and is learning to live, love, and work both as if his days may be short and as if he may live for decades.

Judy's father died when she was thirteen. In her home, she and her two younger siblings were not allowed to talk about their father's death or their feelings about it. Her mother, a college graduate with a business degree, took control of her father's small business. With hard work and long hours, her mother made the business far more successful than it had been before.

For Judy, this was a powerful model of leadership and personal success. At the same time it also meant that she "lost" her mom—in the same way that highly successful corporate executives are often unsuccessful at remaining emotionally close to their children.

When Judy was in high school, her mother married a man who was raising three children by himself. Her mother sold the business and devoted herself to her new blended "Brady Bunch" sort of family. Judy was delighted with her new stepdad and felt happy about the way all six kids knit together and truly felt like siblings.

Judy's stepfather has been her true dad for most of her life and his children became real sister and brothers. She feels blessed and grateful for the events that led to this happening, for the strength and resiliency that came with and through them.

Judy married when she was twenty-one, had three children, and then adopted another. She says that when she adopted a fourth child she could use her experience from her own childhood to handle wanting him to maintain connection with his birth mother, but feeling somehow jealous of his love for her. When she thought back to the way she'd found room in her heart for a "new" dad, she realized that if a mom or dad can love more than one child, then a child can love more than one mom or dad too. With this attitude and feelings of good will, mixed with common sense regarding family roles, she was able to see her son's other mom as a resource, rather than a threat. This led to many positive results for them all.

After twenty years of marriage, Judy and her husband divorced. The divorce was difficult for everyone. However, it created space to bring another family into their lives, just as had happened when she was a teenager. She and her children found that sharing lives and living arrangements with another single-parent family can be very positive. The family that they'd only known slightly before that time has grown into one of the best parts of her family's friendship web. Judy says that through marriages and moves, her large extended family has stayed in close touch.

Judy's professional work includes starting and running a nonprofit organization for single-parent mutual support and home sharing. She says that these are some things she's sure of:

Community is needed in my life.

Most people will be helpful if given a chance.

An assumption of goodwill is an excellent place to begin.

John and Judy wrote this book to provide you with useful and effective guidelines on what to do to create and sustain a network of loving, supportive people. And the good news is that the efforts put into creating your personal safety net and care-sharing team will bring not only safety but also rewards beyond your imagining.

> – Al Siebert, PhD,
> Author of *The Survivor Personality*
> and *The Resiliency Advantage*

Acknowledgments

To the countless individuals and families I have been fortunate to get to know through my professional work, I will be forever grateful.

To the many family members and friends I am blessed to have as a part of my life and whose ongoing love and care sharing provides riches in my life beyond anything I could have imagined, I thank you.

To the many mentors and colleagues, Bonnie Genevay, Wendy Lustbader, Marty Richards, Rick Meyer, Denise Klein, Dr. Albert Wettstein, Kevin Host, Patricia Valdez, Mary Lynn Pannen, and Bonnie Brown Hartley, to name only a few: I am thankful for the opportunity to learn from your unique gifts and use of both head and heart.

To my co-author Judy, I am grateful for all I have learned from you in the last thirteen years. Your capacity to be thoughtful amidst strong emotion and to hold many complexities in your mind and weigh them individually and collectively has taught me much. And above all, your consistent friendship and intellectual integrity has inspired me.

– Dr. John Gibson

Writing this book has been a work of love. It has grown out of my family: both the family of my birth and that of my heart. Dad and Vivian, Kate and Dave, Mary and Roger, Pete and Deborah, Frank and Chris, Michael and Ginny, Brad and Judi, Pam and Rich— thanks to each of you for all the love and lessons in teamwork. To each of my children, Stephan, Cari, Sean, and Damien, I want to say thank you for giving me the opportunity to love you and to learn from you.

Abundant thanks go to my mother, Virginia Helsell, and to Denise Boyd, Todd Hara, Wairimu Kiambuthi, and Marijo Reinhard—all have helped me with big lessons in working together. Bill Helsell has assisted greatly in teaching with love how to step back from a situation to gain a neutral view. It's been amply demonstrated that there is enough love to go around and spill over the edges of the container of our hearts.

Zapote Raphael and Trudy James have contributed to both my education and to this book as teachers, mentors, and friends. Without their exposure to care-team work I'd not have had a context within which to write. Trudy's encouragement and input particularly have immeasurably improved this work.

Anna Kemper Wollenweber has a special place in my heart. She has supported me intellectually and emotionally as I've learned about and participated in care-share teams.

Thanks, too, to the numerous people who have read the manuscript as it's progressed, giving feedback, endorsements, and encouragement.

Lastly, I have overflowing gratitude to John Gibson for being a wonderful person with whom to work.

– Judy Pigott

Together, we particularly want to thank our publisher Elliott Wolf. He came very highly recommended, and his wisdom and guidance met our high expectations at every point along this journey. From the very beginning his support and belief in the importance and value of our book made our many revisions easier and helped us push forward.

Special thanks must be extended to Ruth Kletchka for tirelessly typing what must have seemed like hundreds of drafts. Her timely, excellent work and always-pleasant manner was a joy for us.

Special acknowledgment to our editor, Karen Parkin, who has been a true master of her craft, and whose honesty and competence have been just perfect for the task at hand.

We also extend our thanks to David Marty, Amy Vaughn, Sean Boyd, Colleen Haiber, and all who helped in the production and promotion of our book.

Introduction

This is a book about building community. We believe that one important form community can take is that of a safety net. Many social service agencies and nonprofit organizations provide valuable community safety nets. But we believe it's equally valuable for each of us to intentionally create a personal safety net made up of those resources and individuals who strengthen our lives.

What does it mean to create a personal safety net? It's the process of building caring relationships with people you know want to "be there" for you. As you build and openly value these relationships, you create a sense of security, knowing you have them there for you and you will be there for them. Together, whenever there is a need, you will form a care-share team to address it.

There are many ways you can "be there" for someone else and they, in turn, can "be there" for you. They can simply care about, love, and protect you. They can step in to do for you what you need or want but can't do on your own. Or they can direct you to diverse resources, both practical and emotional, when you need them. Feeling alone or unsupported in a time of need builds fear and anxiety that is damaging on a personal, family, and community level. But the security that having a personal safety net provides reduces fear and anxiety and thereby strengthens individuals, families, and communities.

Some people do not have anything in their lives that even remotely resembles a safety net. Others have a very conscious and explicit group of people that they could quickly call upon. Most of us fall somewhere in between these two extremes. Most of us don't think about safety nets until we've "taken a fall"—when a change or crisis threatens to overwhelm us or someone we love. That's precisely why we've written this book: to encourage you to create a personal safety net before an acute need arises.

> This book will speak to you whether you are experiencing a life change or crisis, or deciding that you want to help someone who is.

This book will speak to you whether you are experiencing a life change or crisis, or deciding that you want to help someone who is. As you read on, you'll discover many stories about people with whom we've worked, people we've loved and cared for, people whose stories we've been told. We have changed the names of individuals—and certain details— to protect their privacy. These stories of real people with real problems will inspire you as you figure out what to do in your own situation. Your challenge is to determine what will work best for you and to make your own decisions. At times, it's hard to know where to begin: You may have doubts, concerns, or uncertainties. Before you take action, you may want to consider seeking a professional assessment and recommendation—this is often time and money well spent.

In addition to the many true stories, this book contains tools, examples, knowledge, and hope to help you make the most of your challenge. God willing, your situation and circumstances will be temporary and you or your loved one will recover. Then you will likely discover that you've developed closer relationships with those who've pitched in, who've become a part of your personal safety net, and who've shared this difficult part of your journey.

> The challenges, joys, and rewards of forming your personal safety net, complete with a care-share team,

If your injury, illness, disability, or challenge is ongoing, then you may find—as we have—that the challenges, joys, and rewards of forming your personal safety net, complete with a care-share team, will lessen the difficulties.

GET READY

Ask yourself:	Is this a book for me?
List:	Who else might benefit from reading this?
Decide:	Should I read this book with a group? And discuss the ideas?

CHAPTER 1

Understand Personal Safety Nets

Your child gets sick and you not only can't drive car pool, but you also can't even see how to get to work. An appointment with your boss turns out to be because you've lost your job. A Saturday walk in the woods brings with it a broken leg. In each case, large or small in scope, you could benefit from the help of a few others. Knowing you have plans, systems, and people who will "cover your back" is what we call a *personal safety net*. Part of this safety net, a crucial part for most of us, is the personal part. And the folks who step in to do the things we cannot do for ourselves are called the *care team* or the *care-share team*. Part of personal success is the ability to invite others into your circle, to allow them to help, and to see strength in creating a team. The team is an integral part of a personal safety net.

WHAT IS A CARE-SHARE TEAM?

A care-share team, then, is an organized group of people who purposefully come together to care for someone in need. This intentional "family" provides for the needs of a family member, a friend, a co-worker, or another individual. A care-share team could just as easily be called a "family of the heart" or "family of choice," that is, a group of people who are acting as if they were relatives. When you create your own personal safety net, then the members "sign up" to be sort of like family to you—and you to them.

Being part of a care-share team enriches the lives of not only the person receiving care but also those who provide it. Participation is typically voluntary, though by necessity participation may be thrust upon an unwilling family member or may include paid professionals. Each person in the care-share team—whether a family member, a friend, a co-worker, a church member, a hired professional, a neighbor, an outside volunteer, or, of course, the care receiver (or *care partner*)—offers his or her own unique gifts.

We intentionally use the term *care partner*, rather than care receiver, to emphasize the giving and receiving of care as a partnership. As illustrated powerfully in Mitch Albom's best-seller *Tuesdays with Morrie*, those on the receiving end of care can give back in many ways. The person receiving care can acknowledge and value that support in a way that makes the most difficult situation better. (Or he could create a living hell for all those who try to help.) At the same time, the person giving care can gain knowledge, experience, and compassion, and, with time, become an even better care-share team member.

But when a team comes together in an organized way to meet different needs, then no one feels the burden of shouldering all the care alone.

The care-share team's goal is to create an environment in which team members can perform at their best and complement each other's efforts. Working together, members support, both practically and emotionally, the care partner—and one another. This may include visiting, transporting, organizing birthday parties and outings, phone calling, taking care of children, doing light housework, grocery shopping, praying, scheduling or going to doctors' appointments, listening, touching, and doing anything else the team and care partner agree upon. The team can brainstorm ways to handle unexpected issues, learn from each other's experiences, offer support in maintaining boundaries (or setting limits), and keep a sense of humor and love.

In situations where there is one primary caregiver, that person often feels alone, overwhelmed, and guilty for not meeting all of the care partner's needs. But when a team comes together in an organized way to meet different needs, then no one feels the burden of shouldering all the care alone. The team significantly lightens the load of the primary caregiver and uncovers what each is willing and able to do. By demonstrating their caring attitude through their presence and actions, team members can encourage their care partner and each other to recognize their own power, to accept themselves and their situation, and to find hope. A high level of trust is likely to develop. All can learn, grow, and deepen connections.

Trust builds out of a sense of caring and understanding. Key to this process is carefully listening to the care partner and other team members without judgment. During difficult times, personal and long-standing issues often rear their ugly heads. Care-share teams agree to avoid preaching, changing, or trying to fix their care partner or each other. They meet regularly for planning and mutual support. Coordinating these meetings can be difficult, since presumably, everyone leads busy lives. However, by working together, each team member can make a difference even with limited time. Most find that participation brings satisfaction, blessings, surprises, and rewards.

Nuns to the Rescue

A young couple with two small children had separated, leaving the mother to care for the children while entering her medical internship. She fretted over how to care for them with required nights on call. Her family lived far away and was unable to help. Her mother in particular worried about how her daughter and grandchildren would handle this challenge. She and her daughter devised a plan.

The young mother went to her church community with an explanation of her problem. Support came from a surprising quarter. Several nuns in the church pooled their available time and skills to form a care-share team. Each time the mother was on call, a rotating member of the team would come in and stay with or pick up the children and care for them until their mom came home. With the team's assistance, the mother handled all of her medical responsibilities and the children were lovingly cared for by their care-share team. The intern's family gained an extended family and the community ultimately gained an empathetic medical practitioner.

WHEN IS A CARE-SHARE TEAM NEEDED?

A care-share team is needed whenever you or someone you love encounters a period, a situation, a predicament, an accident, or a dilemma that would be made better by enlisting help. In the story below, Tony needed a team because he'd run out of ideas, but not out of problems.

Tony Calls Up a Finance-Savvy Team

For years Tony had been trying to get his business to run predictably in the black, but the challenges—being in a cyclical market, offering his services at a discount to friends, neglecting to bill for hours worked and undervaluing his own competencies—kept him from making a profit. A breakthrough came when one of Tony's respected associates suggested he call together several other finance-savvy folks to brainstorm ideas for confronting Tony's business challenges.

Over the next few months, Tony addressed the barriers, one by one. One associate helped manage the billing, another assisted Tony in drafting responses to requests for discounted work. When it was time to face big questions, the group would meet together and discuss suggestions until they found a solution Tony could live with. His finances took a decided upturn, and a time came when he could help others who were starting out on their own business ventures.

These stories demonstrate that the purpose of the care team is to provide for the care partner's health, emotions, psyche, and security. When the whole team stays focused on this purpose, it increases the likelihood that everyone will have a positive feeling about the work. The above stories also show that care-share teams start for many reasons. They can exist for a short time, until someone no longer needs help, or for years.

Paul Shares His Secret

A few years ago, Paul began to notice his golf game deteriorating on the last few holes. It took time for him to relate this to the pain in his feet. His buddies, all in their late forties, could comfortably walk eighteen holes. Paul began to find excuses not to play. It never occurred to him to tell the guys about his arthritis and its growing impact on his life, or to even suggest renting a cart instead of walking the course.

In a way Paul was fortunate. His wife, Jennie, learned about care-share teams and the importance of personal safety nets for hard times when her best friend, Kathy, was diagnosed with breast cancer. She and Kathy had struck up a friendship when their kids started preschool. For years they had shared car pooling and other child-related activities and events. When Kathy's diagnosis came, Jennie joined her care-share team and, over time, learned through trial and error as well as talking with other women in similar situations much about creating a supportive circle of friends.

Paul enjoyed the company of a good friend who loved

to fly-fish. It was when he casually mentioned to Jennie that he might skip their annual fly-fishing trip to Montana that she decided to help Paul do something. She knew it was a mistake for him to start cutting out of his life the things he loved most.

Jennie asked Paul out for a dinner date, saying she had something important to discuss. He was a little alarmed, but she reassured him it was about something important, but good. He relaxed a little. As they talked, Paul forced himself to keep an open mind and listen to Jennie. After all, he had seen how Jennie and her friends had helped Kathy when she needed it; perhaps he could be open to receiving help, too. Even while he admitted to himself that he did need help, he fought the powerful, though subtle, feelings of fear, vulnerability, shame, and uncertainty. Finally, Paul simply said, "Jennie, you're right. I need help and I've been scared and denying it." Jennie tearfully leaned over and gave Paul a big kiss, whispering, "One of the many reasons I've loved you all these years is you've got guts, and another is that you'll listen to me."

That night Jennie and Paul composed an e-mail to all their friends. They explained Paul's arthritis and how it was beginning to impact his life. They invited friends to a potluck, where they could all talk about forming a team to support both of them.

Today, although Paul's arthritis has grown somewhat worse and he is bothered by pain, he regularly golfs (using a *golf cart) and fly-fishes (with a floating device). He admits he has grown closer to many of his friends. While Paul and Jennie sometimes fear what lies ahead, they find strength and comfort in knowing they are not alone. Together they have discovered the unexpected gifts that come from sharing hardship with special friends. As Paul puts it, "Hey, if you want to fly, it's good to have a safety net."*

SPECIFIC CARE-SHARE TEAMS

Whether you're launching a new business, repositioning an existing one onto more solid footing, discovering that you're ill, or going into a divorce, putting a safety net into the equation can ease your feelings of hopelessness, isolation, or fear. But safety nets don't simply *happen*. Neither do care-share teams. You'll need to put some thought and work into constructing a team and aligning both people and resources toward your goal, whether it's finding temporary support for a recovery from illness or surgery; assisting a friend through a degenerative disease to her final days; or building life-long

> Putting a safety net into the equation can ease your feelings of hopelessness, isolation, or fear.

relationships that outlast childcare needs, employment issues, or divorces.

Thirteen Years with No Sign of Stopping

Thirteen years ago, Theo and Eve and their friends Tina and Susan were co-workers getting to know one another. One by one they left their parent company for various reasons, yet stayed in touch. When Theo and Eve moved to a new home, they invited their friends for a housewarming party. During the course of that evening, Tina explained that she was going through a rough patch in her marriage, heading toward divorce, as it turned out. Susan empathized and confessed she was struggling to find the right fit for her career. Both expressed an interest in having a safe and supportive group behind them as they tackled the next steps in their lives. The four agreed to gather the following week, and the week after that, until their gatherings evolved into weekly potlucks at Theo and Eve's house.

Tina's and Susan's problems didn't last forever, but over the years the dinners continued. From time to time the original four friends invited other friends, sometimes to add support, sometimes to receive support, sometimes to add their perspective. There is now a sort of base group of seven or eight.

This group of friends built a kind of safety net,

supporting each other through difficult career moves, starting and closing businesses, divorces and marriages, and caring for elderly parents. All of these difficulties have been held gently by the group as they've sorted out issues, clarified values, prioritized steps, and supported one another.

To this day Theo and Eve's no-longer-new home is the site of these cherished weekly dinners—even when the owners are not home. Starting with a housewarming party, it's matured into a truly warm sort of house of healing where tears and laughter flow.

As you think about forming a care-share team, consider the relationships in your life: Who will be most supportive in this circumstance? Who is the best networker? Who has creative ideas? Who is dependable?

We've found that most teams are formed around the family or the workplace. If you are part of a traditional family, you may choose to include your family members in the care-share team, or you may not. If you live far away from your family, have only a few living relatives, or are otherwise disconnected from family, then thinking more broadly and inviting a different set of people may prove to be more helpful to you.

Throughout this book you'll read many stories of care-share teams comprised mostly of family members. But we also recognize that it may be better for you to choose other people to make up your safety net. In the following story told by a professional care manager, a group of co-workers came together on behalf of their colleague. It could just have well been in a church congregation, school, gym, or neighborhood.

Connie's Co-Workers Step In

The director of human resources called me and asked if we could meet. She explained that a manager in her late thirties, Connie, had early onset Alzheimer's disease. Connie had no family nearby, but her colleagues thought the world of her and wanted to help. First the human resources director and I met with Connie. A few days later, all three of us gathered with interested colleagues to explore how a care-share team could benefit Connie.

In this meeting, it became evident that Connie had a very best friend, Lisa, who was motivated to play a lead role in creating and maintaining a team. As a professional, I could provide examples and connect Lisa with resources. She willingly became the hub of this team. Lisa and other colleagues provided ongoing care. And they involved Connie in decision making—to the extent possible—as well as supported and nourished the involvement of other friends, a boyfriend, and a distant parent. A few other professionals and I provided emotional and physical care in an arrangement that lasted for over six years.

We have observed that there is often concern and caring in the work place when a colleague is ill or has a major life change. Co-workers are often the first to recognize a need. Some work settings are, in turn, more helpful than others in fostering such arrangements. What is often lacking, however, is a leader to guide these well-intended colleagues so that, together, they provide effective care. In the

> Co-workers are often the first to recognize a need.

above example, first the director of human resources and then a paid professional supported Connie's best friend, Lisa, in her role as team leader. Pat Hughes, in *Gracious Space,* wrote that when people join their gifts together, "Individuals improve the quality of their relationships, groups learn to value the different talents and perspectives of their members, and whole organizations and communities become continuous learners, applying mutual respect and creativity to some of their most intractable problems." This is exactly what happens when care-share teams are thoughtfully created.

Johnny Tried to Catch a Piano

Eleven-year-old Johnny never questioned whether he could

catch the piano as he and Freddy rounded the corner much too quickly and it toppled over. The sound could be heard throughout the community center, and their group's rehearsal for the Christmas play came to an abrupt end. Johnny escaped without permanent injury, but did suffer severely cut fingers and bruises on his hands and one foot. Because he couldn't use crutches without two hands he needed a wheel chair, which he also couldn't move by himself because of his bandaged hands.

Johnny's mom, Susan, a single parent with two younger kids and a full-time job, was overwhelmed. An independent and proud woman, Susan didn't think to ask for help. Luckily Jody, one of the other mothers involved in the Christmas play, had great people-organizing skills, which she applied to her family's community, school, and religious activities. She saw Susan's need, recognized that Susan lacked experience in organizing a team, and realized that Susan would probably never ask for help.

Jody asked Susan if she could talk with her. Over a cup of tea she explained her own experience with organizing people. She gently but firmly insisted that Susan let her set up a team of kids and grown-ups to help the family until Johnny recovered. Jody said she missed working as an organizer and it would be fun for her, adding, "Please Susan, let me help." Susan was won over, the group was formed, and Johnny and his family received much-needed support. When Johnny recovered,

Susan even hosted a "pot lunch" to thank all who had helped. Many of the grown-ups were so impressed by what Jody had created that they vowed they would do the same thing if ever there was a need.

Almost anyone who wants to can be part of a care team, if welcomed by the care partner. Intention and commitment are important, as are kindness, flexibility, and the ability to work with others while letting go of control. It's a tall order, but it has been proven that care team participation can include all types of people. Team members will ideally give of what they have, and whatever they bring is sufficient.

We do advise you to use caution and trust your intuition, however, in accepting help from a casual acquaintance or someone who isn't well known to someone in your group (perhaps a new neighbor or a person you've recently talked with in your neighborhood park). It's reasonable to be concerned about safety, especially when your care partner is feeling vulnerable. Some care-share team members we know have gotten background checks from the state police or asked for personal references. If in doubt, take sensible measures to ensure your care partner's security.

> Team members will ideally give of what they have, and whatever they bring is sufficient.

Who's In and Who's Out?

Tina chose to involve a small, consistent nucleus in her care-share team: a dear friend, a paid case manager, a family member, and a counselor-consultant. At various times one of Tina's children, several neighbors, a couple of former colleagues, and a church-related contact all participated. Somewhat surprisingly, no other family members—not even Tina's husband—were included. We never knew the reasons for Tina's selection of care-share team members, but respected and honored her right to exercise preference and control.

So, whether the safety net is for you or someone you know and care about, if it includes a care-share team the crucial element is that it be helpful. It will need a leader and a vision. It will need good will and communication. If you think that shaping a care-share team is absolutely what you need to do, it's time to think it through (which we'll cover in

If this task seems daunting, take heart. You can do it, and do it successfully.

Chapter 2) and consider the people you might want to pull together (more about that in Chapter 3). If this task seems daunting, take heart. You can do it, and do it successfully.

GET READY

Ask yourself: Is there someone in my life (maybe me) who needs help?

List: What can I do for someone else if I'm asked? Make a list of things you think you might do and note whether these are easy or hard for you.

Make another list: Who would I ask if I needed help right now? Do I live in a community where I have strong ties to others? What family help would I want? Start this list.

Decide: Could I benefit from thinking more about who I would turn to if I needed help? Or, if I don't have strong ties that quickly come to mind, do I know anyone who I think could help me brainstorm ideas? Who?

Compile: Gather names and numbers for the legal and financial parts of your life. This part of your safety net can be put into place now and updated every few years.

CHAPTER 2
Think It Through

Before you enter a care-share relationship—whether you need help or want to offer help—it's important to think through basic needs and values, examine your own motivations, and ask yourself if your life will be enhanced by enlisting help from or offering assistance to others.

BASIC INTERPERSONAL HUMAN NEEDS

All humans have a basic need to be in relationship with significant others. It is life enhancing to share feelings, needs, hopes, and fears— and in so doing develop a trust and security with another person. All humans have a basic need to be recognized and valued. This helps create and sustain a unique and valuable sense of self. All human beings have a need to nurture and to be nurtured, to receive care and to give care. Expressing concern, perceiving that concern is

> **All human beings have a need to nurture and to be nurtured, to receive care and to give care.**

received, and accepting the care and love of another contribute to a deep sense of well-being.

When someone is ill or during a major life change, it becomes even more important for these basic interpersonal human needs to be met. However, this happens while one's time, energy, and power are compromised. Both care partners and team members need to actively try to recognize and meet their own and the other's needs.

In the following story, a family demonstrates their ability to meet each other's needs during great adversity. Their common values of openness, gratitude, and caring helped ten-year-old Mario to grow up with resiliency and hope despite being part of a family that was encountering multiple and serious challenges.

When Will I Lose My Hair, Mommy?

"When will I lose my hair?" he asked Linda, his mom. Mario was ten years old when his nineteen-year-old sister discovered she had cancer of the brain. He was ten when his mother's ovarian cancer was diagnosed and eleven when she finished extensive chemotherapy for her cancer that had metastasized. She was given only a 5 percent chance of living one year. That same year, Mario's grandpa received treatments for prostate cancer. And all had lost hair during treatments. Mario's mom smiled at her son's question and said she didn't think he would ever

lose his hair.

Amid their tragedies, the family remained open and loving. All members were doing much better than expected. Their friends and other relatives formed a strong care-share team that included Mario and his dad, Walt. This had paid off. Mario took pride in helping his mommy and big sister. Walt continued working without having to take much time off, which helped with the enormous medical bills.

What's more, the care team wrote a vision statement that pulled them together and guided their decisions. Life wasn't all smooth sailing, but it did progressively become calmer.

Linda and Walt expressed gratitude for the care-sharing team. The team members themselves were grateful. The depth of the family's tragedy and trauma had touched and even blessed each one. Each took life and health much less for granted. They were all forever changed by the love and resilience they witnessed and shared. Finally, each team member knew that he or she had truly made a difference in the lives of the family.

There is an old saying that God gave us two hands: one to receive with and one to give with. This means we are not made for hoarding our time, talent, or treasure, rather, we are channels made for sharing. Mario's family really understood the power of this truth. They weren't afraid of asking for—or giving or receiving—help.

ENTERING NEW TERRITORY

Asking for help. Giving help. Saying yes, saying no. Feeling uncertain. Not knowing what to expect. Not wanting to over commit. Not wanting to disappoint. These are some of the thoughts, fears, and dilemmas you face when you are seriously challenged, ill, or when you are "up close" to someone who is seriously ill.

How do I feel? How will I feel? Will those who will help me feel shame, uncertainty, anxiety, tenderness, embarrassment, and anger like I do? What if I lose it and break down? What if they lose it and break down? What if they're not there? What if they can't do it? What if they really want to help, but I can't bring myself to ask? The questions and unknowns are endless.

Life's inevitable challenges and changes thrust us into new territory. We invite you to enter this territory with humbleness,

> We are not made for hoarding our time, talent, or treasure, rather, we are channels made for sharing.

for surely it will humble you. We invite you to view every encounter as an opportunity to grow. Surely, we all know very little and need to learn more for this journey. This may be the right time for you to come to trust a personal friend or a professional counselor who can help you sort things out. Draw upon the collective wisdom by including others to inform and guide you through the difficult parts of your life journey.

WHAT IS IT LIKE TO BE SICK?

Any illness, especially a life-threatening illness, has emotional impact much like a large rock dropped into the middle of a lake. It sends a powerful ripple through the lives of family and friends. They may experience feelings, thoughts, and reactions they've never felt before, which may overwhelm or frighten them. Surprisingly, an illness may even sometimes produce peaceful and reassuring feelings, especially if people step in to help, or if inner work is prompted. Illness always impacts relationships, often in unanticipated ways—sometimes welcome, sometimes not.

> Any illness, especially a life-threatening illness, has emotional impact much like a large rock dropped into the middle of a lake. It sends a powerful ripple.

Facing a life-threatening illness may stir within you important questions about the meaning of life and what really matters. It also presents an opportunity for you to look deep within and review and reformulate your values, hopes, fears, and beliefs.

In this journey into new and unknown territory, you may feel your innocence is lost, your life suppositions shaken. You may feel vulnerable, not knowing what, when, why, or how. People close to you may seem to be going about their lives as if nothing has changed, yet for you everything is different. You've crossed a line between health and illness, and now you see everything from a different lens.

RECEIVING CARE IS AN ART

We believe receiving care is an art that few of us learn in our lifetime. In our three decades of personal and professional involvement with people facing serious challenges, we have met only a few who seemed at ease with being on the receiving end of care. We encourage you to *practice* the healthy attitudes listed below at every opportunity. If you're aware of these qualities when you face minor illnesses or the normal disruptions of starting a new endeavor, then when challenged by the bigger ones, you will know well the territory of receiving care. Begin by thinking about these statements and their truth in your life today.

- I am comfortable with needing help.

- I can recognize and ask for what I need, not more than what I need. I am not overly reliant on others. I also avoid asking for less than what I need and thereby suffering unnecessarily.

- When someone helps me, I feel grateful, not guilty, embarrassed, or shamed.

In the book *Tuesdays with Morrie*, the main character, Morrie, is suffering from a progressive neurological disorder. This will slowly render him unable to care for himself. He knows this and strives to learn, as the disease progresses, to receive in a gracious, pleased, and grateful way. He hopes that people who care for him, after feeding him, or grooming him, or even in his worst nightmare, as he put it, "wiping his ass," will somehow feel they've given him a precious gift. He hopes that he has received that gift in such a way that those who've helped him will have that wonderful feeling inside them that we all get after we've given someone the perfect gift.

Whatever your change or challenge may be, it's our hope that you'll be able to feel good about asking for, giving, or receiving care. In what may be one of the biggest challenges of all, the beloved minister and columnist Rodney R. Romney wrote the following words of gratitude for the role he'd unknowingly played for his brother.

Facing Your Own Death

A few months ago in this column I wrote about "Making

Friends with Our Own Death." Little did I then realize that I would soon be faced with the challenge of making friends with the death of a member of my immediate family. My brother, Dick, died on July 18 after a brief but intensive bout with cancer.

We had gathered as a family around his bedside in a hospital room, where he had been struggling for several weeks, when he looked at me and said weakly, "I am tired of this and ready to go. Please pray for me." I held his hand and prayed that God would bless him and all of us as we learned to let go of life and entrust it into the hands of the One who had created us. As my prayer ended, I felt his hand relax in mine. Within a few minutes, he was gone. I watched the light of life fade from his eyes and felt his heart rate slow down and eventually cease. In the aftermath of that experience, I realized it is sometimes easier to accept our own death than it is to accept the death of a loved one.

This brother was a person who had a great love for nature and its creatures. He had never manifested any interest in organized religion and avoided formal religious services whenever he could. Still, he was religious in his own way, finding his strength in nature and the outdoors rather than in a church. By contrast, I had spent most of my adult life as a minister planning and conducting all kinds of religious services. Yet in those final moments of his life, we were equal, both seeking comfort and guidance from the unknown and unseen force of life.

Several days after his death, as we sorted through his belongings, I discovered that he had kept a laminated copy of my column on making friends with death. I realized then that he must have found meaning in my words, for he had died with peace and total acceptance of the fact that his life was over. I can only hope that when my own moment of departure comes, I will enter into it with as much trust as he had shown.

When you are prepared for what's ahead, the future is much easier to face. Often, though, you must meet what's difficult, scary, or unknown before the preparation begins. Illness, injury, and major life changes (even our own death or that of a loved one) come by surprise. Often those who are involved know little if anything about what the care partner is experiencing. Preparing to face the future includes learning about the illness or change, mapping out the possible scenarios and probable journey, and finding out what skills, knowledge, and resources you may need. If you can accept that you are a beginner in this new and often unexpected and unwanted change in life, and move forward as a student, rapid learning will follow. With this will come a sense of stability and control, which will, in turn, decrease anxiety. Replacing resistance with curiosity will diminish your fears.

> If you can accept that you are a beginner in this new and often unexpected and unwanted change in life, and move forward as a student, rapid learning will follow.

Recruiting and involving friends, associates, and relatives for your journey will immeasurably enrich all your lives.

CASTING A SAFETY NET

Is the life change you are going through serious enough to seek out more resources or ask others for help? If you are thinking that it's time to answer this question, then you're ready to get started. Ask yourself the questions below—whether you are experiencing a challenge in your own life or are considering entering into someone else's scenario. The answers may not come easily. In fact, prepare to initially want to contradict yourself or to reject your own answers: They can be difficult to accept. However, planning for the worst-case scenario also prepares you for a variety of situations as well as opportunities to make your life better despite the changes and challenges.

SHOULD I START A CARE-SHARE TEAM?

1. Is my life getting beyond my control?

2. Do I find it hard to take care of myself? Think of cooking, shopping, bathing, taking medications (getting them, remembering to take them, coordinating and distinguishing them), staying in touch with loved ones, telephoning, paying bills or managing finances, housekeeping, taking care of children and their needs, transportation, and many other daily tasks.

3. Are there people, paid or unpaid, who are helping me or might if asked?

4. Am I lonely?

5. Am I isolating myself?

6. Are the people who are helping me acting as if they're tired or burdened?

7. Do I wish I had the answers to more questions about how to handle various aspects of living with my condition? Think of health, finances, insurance, etc.

8. Has something changed?

Write out your answers to these questions without judging the answers or strategizing the solution. (We will get to that later.)

Bill Cries, "I Lost My Wife"

Bill and Alice were happily married for sixty-two years. They cared for each other and relished their independence. They also enjoyed a close relationship with their two sons who lived and worked in the same city, and a daughter who lived three hours away. When Alice began to develop forgetfulness and balance problems, the family attributed this to normal aging. As symptoms worsened, however, it became clear that her ability to function normally was rapidly deteriorating. Alice was diagnosed with Alzheimer's disease. Bill was distraught. "I've lost my wife," he thought.

Bill was capable of caring for himself and wanted desperately to help Alice. But as her condition deteriorated, he became more and more tired and depressed. When Alice began to fall and her memory worsened, he worried constantly about her. He doubted his ability to continue being there for her. It was clear that more help or a team was needed to aid Alice as well as to ensure that Bill's own fragile health was not compromised.

Bill's sons noticed the obvious strain on their father. Because Alice's condition was rapidly declining, none of them knew what to expect. Meanwhile, Bill was exhausting himself and isolating himself from his other interests, activities, and friends. He was devoting all of his time, attention, and care to his wife and their home. His family knew this was dangerous. His daughter in-law, who had participated in a tele-video course called "You and Your Aging Parents," suggested that Bill seek professional help. He agreed.

Bill and his sons met with the counselor, who asked, "What are you doing now? What can your friends do? Have you asked any of them? Can you afford paid help and would it be accepted?"

They acknowledged the current efforts of all the family members. They agreed that some support for both Alice and Bill was well in place, but they still needed more help, which they could divide among family or friends. Two granddaughters, who were high school age and needed spending money, agreed to do some of the household chores and grocery shopping. Their grandpa was happy to pay them, *and, more importantly, delighted to spend some enjoyable moments with his two bubbly, energetic granddaughters.*

The family hired a home-health agency to help monitor and treat the diabetes that Alice had recently developed. Agency aides also helped with morning and nighttime bathing, grooming, and dressing. One of the sons developed a list of his parents' friends, including names, addresses, phone numbers, and e-mail addresses. With the blessing of his dad, his son sent out an appeal for help, informing their family and friends of Alice's situation. People stepped in to spend time with Alice, accompany her on walks, go through photographs, and simply be with her during mealtimes so that Bill could spend some time on the golf course.

The care-share team they developed was a blessing to Bill as he not only resumed his normal activities but also received constant encouragement and support. As Alice's disease, dementia, and disability worsened, the team grew.

At first it's often easy to think you can manage any situation or beloved care partner by yourself and avoid asking for help. However, again we urge you to consider asking. First ask yourself the questions from the above list, as Bill's counselor urged him and his family to do. Then, with the added insight these answers will bring, either begin to take action or seek assistance in doing so. There is much to be gained for yourself and a care partner through creating a personal safety net—a team—to share in the care.

With these questions answered, you've taken the first step to solving the problem. Now you are better equipped to explain to your care-share team what you need and how they might help. You are beginning to create a plan.

As you read on, keep asking yourself how you can modify a care plan to improve life during this difficult time. If you create or join a care-share team you will be maintaining a fine balance of independence, dependency, and engaging in a lot of honest but sensitive communication. Remember, the care partner is in control but needs to use his influence with tact and respect.

> Remember, the care partner is in control but needs to use his influence with tact and respect.

The following story tells how Ron had to search his own heart and answer big questions before he was ready to reach out to friends for the help he needed. They, in turn, had to ask themselves if they were ready to say yes.

Ron Takes the Step and Asks

Ron, a 68-year-old former stockbroker, suffered a small stroke that left his right side partially paralyzed. His condition was stable but required a hospital stay, and his long-term prognosis was uncertain. To make matters worse, Ron was still grieving his wife, who had died eight months earlier, and depending upon his daughter, Julia, to help him both emotionally and practically. Now during his hospital stay, Ron didn't want to burden Julia any further. His neurological function was improving, but things were piling up at home. He knew he needed help, but whom to ask and how?

Years earlier, Ron and a group of his friends had made a pact, a promise that if anyone got in trouble, each would be there to help. When Ron made this pact, he had assumed he would be the first to offer, not to ask for, assistance. He was accustomed to remaining silent about health-related problems but he knew he needed to tell his friends of his dilemma. That was their promise to each other. As he prepared to call his "pact" friends, he thought about his wife and how much she had needed him at the end. "Is this my end?" he thought. He missed her now more than ever and wished she were still alive to help him. "She knew me, knew what I needed. She took care of me! I know now what she might have felt."

It was painful for Ron to ask for help outside of his family. "The Korean War was easier than this," he mused. "But I have to do it." With courage and a sense of responsibility to his friends, he called each of them and explained that he'd had a stroke and was in the hospital. Every friend, without *exception, asked, "Is there anything I can do?" He replied, "Yes, but I will need your help to figure out exactly what needs to be done and to help organize my recovery."*

Ron's taking the risk of asking for help was step one in his new plan. It proved to be a good one. Not only he, but also his daughter, benefited greatly from his courage to ask. Ron's friends stepped up during his recovery: Together they developed and continued to modify a plan that changed as Ron became stronger. They valued his friendship and appreciated him for many things, including his years of military service during the Korean War and his model of how strength could mean enlisting help.

LOOK AT YOUR MOTIVATIONS

Have you asked yourself *why* you want to help? Being part of a care-share team may be one way of making a life to be proud of, assuming it is done in a loving and life-giving way. "I'm helping because I can, and I'll enrich my life in the process." "I love this person." "I want to reach out." "This person has done so much for me, I want to give back." Or even, "I'll feel so guilty if I don't." "I didn't help last time, this time I need to do it." These are answers frequently given. There's no particular reason for stepping into a care-share team that's better or more valid than another, but it can be helpful to know why *you* want to do so. Then, if you face a tough period in the life of this team, you'll be able to remember why it is that you said yes. If you are asked why you'd choose to take part in someone else's personal safety net, you'll have an answer. Your answer may even hold some surprises for you.

CLARIFYING QUESTIONS

- Do I want to carry this alone? (I may need help.)
- Am I the only person he/she relies on? Do I want that much responsibility? (Probably not, and a team might help.)
- Am I experiencing burnout? (A team could help me take a breather.)
- Can I meet my own needs during all of this? (Few of us can.)
- Do I have a good perspective on this situation? (Maybe.)
- Am I willing to adjust my life to revolve completely around this person's needs? (If so, how much or in what ways?)
- Would this person's life be better if there were more people assisting?

Beyond congratulating yourself for wanting to help, look at whether you're expecting to make miracles happen, to put off "the inevitable," to feel loved and needed, or to make someone happy. Knowing why you're offering care can help you recognize successes as well as understand frustrations.

In the book *Gracious Space*, Pat Hughes identifies curiosity and compassion as deeper motivations that cause some of us to want to help: "Bring a spirit of compassion and curiosity: compassion for both the vulnerable and less fortunate as well as for ourselves, curiosity from a deep desire to understand, a capacity to engage, and a willingness to shift fundamental beliefs. . . . In deep curiosity we feel driven to get to know others better,

> Being able to set realistic expectations and adhere to them is an essential care-team member skill.

to truly understand where they are coming from and what they can offer to the problem at hand. Deep curiosity is a willingness to hang in there, to seek the gem in another's point of view, even if we don't like the person." Hughes further notes that curiosity and compassion will enhance the lives of both the giver and the receiver. Other motivations such as guilt or a desire for control will not be of much help. But most of us approach a crisis with mixed motives. Becoming clear about your own motivations will help when things get tough.

SET REALISTIC EXPECTATIONS

The ins and outs of caregiving, care receiving, and being part of a care-share team may be new territory for you. Thinking through—and "imaging" through—what this might entail will help you prepare and make better choices. You may begin helping enthusiastically, only to discover the situation is more complex than you anticipated. Being able to set realistic expectations and adhere to them is an essential care-team member skill. As you face each new situation, think through how others might feel and what they might think. See if you can talk about different perspectives: This will help you become a better partner. Finally, if you have the luxury to "think through" what's coming with a trusted friend, relative, or professional, there's the possibility of valuable input.

Megan's Story

Megan and her husband, Hugh, created a care team when she needed surgery. They determined they would need help during the first three to four weeks after Megan's surgery. They began thinking through two difficult questions to identify what needs or "jobs" they would like care-share team members to do.

The first question was, "What are all the things Megan does now that she won't be able to do during her recovery time?" The answer was that Megan did one heck of a lot, which was both good and bad news. The good news was that Hugh now realized how much she did and began to appreciate this more. The bad news was a lot of work would be left to do, unless someone else picked up the pieces. Megan's first thought was that Hugh could handle it all; he could pick up the slack. Hugh, however, had an equally full life, with his own tasks and obligations. He worried about feeling overwhelmed, exhausted, and grouchy, and missing out on spending quality time with her as she recovered.

Then they asked themselves, "What are the things that Hugh normally does that care-share team members might also do?" Hugh wanted to devote time and energy to being present with Megan, giving her his tender-loving care. Together they decided to ask the care-share team to support them by taking over many of Megan's tasks, plus a few of Hugh's responsibilities.

With this in mind, Megan and Hugh made a list of tasks and divided them into these categories: housekeeping, being on call in case Megan needed urgent transportation, occasionally preparing meals, and simply spending time with close friends.

Hugh and Megan pulled together quite a team. In the weeks before her surgery, they prepared by accomplishing the following:

- *Hired a paid housekeeper for some household chores (four hours, twice a week)*
- *Asked neighbors to be "on call" for urgent transportation.*

- *Arranged for friends to bring a few meals and stay with Megan for conversation and companionship on nights when Hugh was gone.*
- *Asked someone to return and pick up videos for Megan to watch.*
- *Invited close women friends to enjoy time with Megan as she used her convalescence to begin creating photo albums for her two children.*

Finally, Hugh used his cell phone and e-mail lists and got busy with his help-appeal script. He set aside an entire evening to call potential care-share team members and let them know of his wife's upcoming surgery. He briefly described some of their needs and asked for help.

He carefully acknowledged that each person had a busy life and simply might not be able to participate. With only a couple of exceptions, their friends and family expressed a desire to help in large or small ways. Delighted and relieved, Hugh got busy organizing this newly formed care-share team via e-mail communication.

When two people have lives that are very intertwined and interdependent, an illness or a life crisis impacts both. Further, if both are working, as is frequently the case, and they share decision making, thinking and talking it through is a major, complicated, and delicate task. Even if it's difficult, sharing care is certainly the better alternative to receiving no help at all.

ASSUME YOU HAVE NEEDS, TOO

Because it's important to consider your own capabilities, needs, and expectations as well as the needs and expectations of your care partner, it's best to enter the care-share situation *presuming* you have needs and *asking* yourself what they are. Clearly and respectfully communicating your needs helps avoid many problems. In Martha's story below, a friend tells how she balanced Martha's needs with her own.

> Enter the care-share situation presuming you have needs and asking yourself what they are.

Martha

I was not the only person Martha called when she needed help: She asked one person to collect mail, another to grocery shop, and another to drive her to doctors' appointments. Because she worked hard to make sure none of us ever met each other, we never did. This arrangement went on for months and months.

Most important to Martha was holding the vision of her

body as strong, healthy, and whole. This was her hope, through a mastectomy, stem cell transplant, metastases, recurring infections, and, finally, pulmonary failure, pneumonia, and death. But if anyone urged her to accept "reality"—the progression of her disease—she considered them unhelpful and dropped them by the wayside, cutting off communication altogether.

What was clear to me was that I could only participate in this unformed "team" if I could suspend disbelief enough to hold Martha's vision of health, mirroring it back to her through thick and thin. This was her life, and I decided I could do this for her. Yet I could only commit a couple of hours a week to her because of the strain this caused me. To do more I would have needed a cohesive team—just what she was avoiding! I gave what I was comfortable with and did that gladly since I stayed within my own comfort zone.

Balancing the needs of the care partner with your needs, as well as those of the other care-share team members, involves getting to know yourself better. (To read more about balancing needs, see Take Care of Yourself in Chapter 5 and Burnout in Chapter 6.)

Now that you've asked yourself the hard questions, examined your values and motivations, and learned a little more about what caregiving and receiving is all about, you're getting ready to take the next important step: Asking others for help. It's not as hard as you think. Read on to discover more.

GET READY

Ask yourself:	What do I value most in life? (Write down your five most important values.)
Think:	Do I believe that relationships with others are important? What are my five deepest relationships? Do I believe that it's important to both give and receive care?
Remember:	When did I help someone out or someone helped me, and it felt good? Was there ever a time when it felt bad? Can I remember why?
Practice:	List the steps needed to tackle any task in front of you, then prioritize them.

CHAPTER 3
Ask for Help

Creating a care-share team from within your safety net requires you—at some point—to ask for help. We call this a *help appeal*. We first learned of help appeal in Zurich, Switzerland, at a lecture given by the author, Dr. John Gibson, and attended by Dr. Albert Wettstein, Switzerland's director of Public Health. Afterward, Dr. Wettstein explained to John that the Swiss, particularly men, are very private and self-reliant, and dreadfully bad about communicating a medical or life problem. Dr. Wettstein said, "I invented help appeal for us Swiss so we could deal much better with illness."

> With a simple script in hand, the men found it much easier to ask for help.

According to Dr. Wettstein, developing help appeal was quite simple. He created sample letters and telephone-call scripts that instructed people how to explain an illness to friends and relatives. Those letters and call scripts became the help appeal that these men (and sometimes women) used to tell their friends and relatives about an illness, disability, disease, or extensive and frightening medical test. With a simple script in hand, the men found it much easier to ask for help. We've found that a similar approach can be equally well applied when facing other life changes and challenges.

Dr. Wettstein added, "You Americans have 'sex appeal.' I watch your TV and see how sex appeal is used to sell everything. Now we Swiss have 'help appeal.'"

Jim's Help-Appeal Phone Call

"Hello," Jim said over the phone to his old friend Fred. "I have something important to tell you. Do you have a couple of minutes? I've just come back from a follow-up visit to my doctor, where I was told, based on the biopsy, that I have prostate cancer. I don't yet know what this will mean for me. I may be cured, maybe not; it may require a lot and be a long ordeal, maybe not. I will find out more in the coming weeks. In the meantime, I wanted you to know. I don't know how you can help me during this time, but just knowing that you are there is helpful to me. I'll keep you posted as I learn more about my cancer and what I have to do. Oh, you should also know that I am not restricted in any of my activities, so we can still go on our Saturday morning walk around the lake and have breakfast afterward."

Jim's example may help you think about drafting your own script. If you have invited others to join you in creating a safety net or forming a care-share team for yourself or someone else, we'd love for you to tell us about it: Go to the Personal Invitation to Readers in the back of the book to find out how. By sharing your experience you will help us create what we hope will be a second book of examples that will serve as encouragement and support for others. You'll be part of creating a written safety net for future readers.

In our years of working with care-share teams, we've discovered many simple, effective ways to ask for help; there's no *one* way that's right for everyone. In the following stories, Sarah, Lisa, Mary, and Sid preferred face-to-face requests and letters to communicate, while Ted and Sue used e-mail and phone calls.

Sarah's Dilemma: Home or Nursing Home?

Sarah, an independent and widowed 71-year-old woman, knew it would be hard to ask for aid after her hip replacement surgery. She also knew that if she didn't have help, she would be forced to spend extra days in a rehabilitation center or nursing home. And she would have to pay for a 24-hour caregiver until she could get around her house, and then for more days, maybe weeks, until she could drive, grocery shop, and go back to her normal life.

Sarah made some notes to herself on how she would express her help appeal to her good friends. With notes completed and words rehearsed, she mustered up her courage and invited her five best friends for a potluck dinner at her house. So that she wouldn't back out at the last minute, she told them that she had something important to say.

When the evening came, Sarah sat down with her friends and began with a simple explanation: "You all are my best friends and I know you have busy lives. I need to have hip replacement surgery, and I'm not sure what all my recovery will entail, but I know I will need help." One of Sarah's younger friends immediately jumped in, "Oh, my aunt went through that and the whole family helped her. We'll be your family. I'll make a list of things you may need. I'll ask my aunt, and we can make a schedule." Another friend offered, "And I can come and sleep here, I'm retired. Laurence [her husband] won't mind, and we can eat popcorn, watch sappy videos, and before you know it you'll be up and around."

Sarah's friends showed that they cared about her in a way that she had not anticipated, and that deeply touched her. These friends, and a few others, instantly formed the care-share team for Sarah that allowed her to go home. This incredibly kind act not only relieved Sarah, but also enriched the lives of all of her friends, who, in turn, became closer to one another.

Ted's E-mail to Warren's High-Tech Work Group

I think all of you know by now that Warren has cancer. There's no cure for it, and the doctors don't give him much of a chance for living through the year.

Doesn't get any tougher. Warren, his wife, Carolyn, and their eight year old will need our help. I watched a cousin go through this a couple of years ago and it's brutal.

Warren and I are close. I've talked with Carolyn, and they're open to help. I'll be lead on this one. Same rules: Don't take on anything you don't think you can do. Communicate, communicate, communicate.

More e-mails shortly. – Ted

His work group's responsiveness pleased Ted. Not everyone could actively participate in the team, but Ted knew that Warren would feel really good about receiving so many expressions of concern.

Ten-year-old Lisa took a straightforward tact in asking for exactly what she needed.

Lisa's Letter to Her Fourth-Grade Classmates

Hi Everybody,

Thank you for your get-well cards. My doctor says I

am getting better fast even though the car wreck was just three days ago. I miss all of you and Miss Brown, too. The doctor doesn't know when I'll be able to go home and back to school. I don't want to get way behind in my classes and maybe fail. Will you help me?

Here is what I know I need now: Miss Brown's notes and assignments for all my classes. Please pick up my library book so I can start my book report. Pick up a video and watch it with me. And visit me on Sunday because my family has to go to Grandma's for her birthday.

Thank you, Lisa

Some situations are far more complicated than Lisa's. When you're faced with a long-term illness or difficult diagnosis, sometimes the only thing you're certain of is that you need help. You may need to gather your team together to figure out how to proceed. That worked well for Tom and Sue in the next story.

Sue Steps In

Tom found out that the symptoms he'd been experiencing were due to an advanced cancer. Overwhelmed at the thought of a foreshortened life, he fell into a deep depression that threatened to flood his partner. Sue, however, had had some experience with illness in her family and decided to reach out on Tom's behalf. Calling on Tom's sister and brother and a cadre of friends, she outlined his diagnosis, the course that they expected him to take, and both of their needs. Most of those contacted were ready to help immediately. Sue set up an initial meeting to define some roles and expectations, and Tom found himself surrounded by loving, caring team members who stood by them during his treatments.

In yet another case of someone seeking help for a spouse, Mary reached out by letter to the couple's church group. Not knowing what might be needed or helpful, Mary simply explained Sid's situation. The responses became the inspiration she needed to later mold a care-share team.

Mary and Sid's Letter to Their Congregation

Dear Friends,

As some of you may know, Sid suffered a major stroke six days ago. The doctors won't say how much he will recover. He will start speech and physical therapy in the coming weeks. We both missed attending church last Sunday and sharing the fellowship of your company.

Sid and I don't know what the coming weeks and months will bring, but we ask you, our friends of many years, to hold us in your prayers, along with the many others who also need your prayers.

Sid has been home for two days, and we're realizing how different our lives will be for the foreseeable future. We don't know yet what help we will need, and we know that many of you are already over committed and over extended. We would absolutely not want to add more to your load, but I can imagine that some assistance would make a big difference in our lives.

Sincerely, Mary and Sid

As Dr. Wettstein had identified for Swiss men, the value was in the *asking* and *receiving*, which is true for all of us. We want to help you integrate the help-appeal concept into your life. We want to help you understand the power of sharing in the care of others. We build and strengthen our personal community through asking for and giving help. This is a radical shift in the definition of strength. We suggest that strength lies in taking control through asking, delegating, and getting ready.

> We build and strengthen our personal community through asking for and giving help.

PRACTICE WILL HELP

It's often not easy to ask for help. The internal muscles required for doing so don't get much exercise in our culture: It takes practice. You can start laying the groundwork for reaching out. Solely for the practice, you can invite neighbors to a potluck, ask for directions, call a friend to join you for a movie, or ask others to join you in forming a volunteer group to support someone else. The important part is to begin practicing both asking for help and giving it.

> The important part is to begin practicing both asking for help and giving it.

Any of these activities, especially if they're unfamiliar, will gently stretch your capacity to reach out. Some version of the words "Is it okay if I ask you for help?" is almost always met with willingness. Even if the person can't do what you had hoped, you've opened a door. And each opening will make it easier to talk about things that are scary or make you feel vulnerable. Getting comfortable asking with relatively simple and small requests is a powerful step toward preparing yourself to ask in a life-changing event. Besides being culturally conditioned to be independent, we face other barriers that keep us from disclosing our needs and requesting assistance.

BARRIERS TO ASKING FOR HELP

Some common barriers that often get in the way of asking for help include these questions and fears:

- "What if they say no?" (a fear factor)
- "I can't ask: In our family we take care of our own." (a pride factor)
- "I don't want to be 'beholden' to anyone." (a self-worth question)
- "I can take care of myself." (an individualist myth)
- "If I ask for help, I'll look weak." (another pride factor)
- "If they really knew me, they'd reject me." (another self-worth question)

Yet, the very same people who voice these fears often describe how good they felt when they've helped a friend or family member. They also admit that giving help and interacting with others while doing so deepens their relationships. Deep down, they know that good things often come from both helping and being helped. In times of stress and need, however, fears and questions can get in the way.

> Granted, asking for help is a risk, but many of the best things in life only come when we reach out and take some risks.

Granted, asking for help is a risk, but many of the best things in life only come when we reach out and take some risks.

Even when you do risk asking for help, there may be times when you don't want to accept the sort of assistance that is offered. In fact, you may have very good reasons for rejecting someone's offer. John was surprised when Peter initially declined his offer, as he tells in this story.

If I Ask, Can I Trust You to Say No?

My neighbor, Peter, recently was diagnosed with cancer. He needed radiation treatments daily. When I found out I asked, "Peter, can I help you move in and out of your wheelchair, take you to your radiation treatments, and help you with any personal physical issues?" He smiled, "John, thanks. I would agree, but you know that I am not sure I can trust you." I was stunned and asked what he meant. He said, "I would only feel free to ask you to help me if I felt confident you would say no if you had something else you really needed to do." His eyes locked into mine and I realized he couldn't be more serious.

As was his way, he sat quietly and patiently while I collected myself. When he saw I was ready to respond he added, "I have had several people sign up to help me. With a couple of them, like you, I've wanted reassurance that they could say no if they needed to. Some couldn't or wouldn't say no when they needed to and it became awkward for both of us. I want you to know that I value your offer, but I am worried that it will affect our relationship."

Peter gave me permission to say no, whenever and without guilt. What a gift! When I promised to say no if I needed to, he knew I meant it. He smiled and said, "I'll put you on my list!" He felt better once he'd gotten over his worry about me. Eventually during my time with him, I occasionally had to say no. Peter laughed each time and said, "So I can trust you, can I! Well, good! Thanks, buddy, for all you've done, and I'll call again soon."

John learned a valuable lesson from his friend: It's important to keep personal commitments and needs in mind when extending help.

BARRIERS TO SAYING "I'LL HELP"

As shown in John's story above, there can be reasons why someone might not be an appropriate person to ask for help. The story also illustrates why someone might be reluctant to offer. We have observed many barriers to saying yes to an appeal for help. Some of the more common barriers include these:

> It's important to keep personal commitments and needs in mind when extending help.

- "What if they ask me to give more than I can right now?" (a question of being able to set limits or boundaries)
- "I won't be able to cut back on or stop helping when I need to." (a fear of being overwhelmed)
- "I can't intrude." (a belief about privacy)
- "This is a family matter. They should handle it themselves." (a myth about independence)
- "I'm uncomfortable around sick people." (a fear of discomfort)
- "My life is already too full." (another fear of being overwhelmed)

Analyze—and perhaps challenge—your fears or concerns. At least start by gathering more information. Look for small ways you can help. In most settings you can discuss concerns and constraints on your availability with the person asking for help.

You may not be accustomed to having this sort of open and honest personal discussion. However, we believe in our increasingly complex world, with increased life expectancy and accompanying periods of illness or disability, we all need to practice and get better at these sorts of conversations. The point is to offer what you can freely give, as Rosa does in this story.

Rosa's Telephone Message to Patricia before Her First Chemo

Hi Patricia, this is Rosa. I know this afternoon is your first chemotherapy. I have been saying prayers for you. I have asked the spirits of my ancestors, guardian angels, and our heavenly father to guide your treatment to the very best outcome. I pray that your heart will swell with the love all of us send to you, make you stronger, and channel the medicines to just where they are needed. We go with you on this day as we will always go with you, but we send a little extra love this morning and throughout the day.

Patricia, we all love you.

IT'S HARD TO ASK

Most people prefer not to have to ask for help. A few recoil at the very idea and can't even imagine asking. For a few it's easy. In between are the many for whom it's difficult or for whom the preceding barriers get in the way, but who determine to go ahead anyway. Learning how to ask for, accept, and offer support is an essential life skill. Asking for help can be an act of love and protectiveness toward those who are loved. Receiving it can be a gift to the giver. The next story tells a little bit of one couple who really understood this.

> Learning how to ask for, accept, and offer support is an essential life skill.

Alfonso's Help Appeal: Update E-mail to His Team

Alfonso, the pillar of good health, was diagnosed with cancer.

He and wife, Lana—through phone calls, in-person conversations, and e-mail messages—notified friends and relatives of his diagnosis. Lana regularly sent out e-mails letting their friends and family know how Alfonso was doing. The latest e-mail described his upcoming chemotherapy and asked that all hold him warmly in their hearts and in their prayers.

You *can* become comfortable with asking for help. With time and practice, you will be able to ask in a calm, easy manner and to receive responses in a levelheaded and thoughtful way. It's not easy to respond calmly in the midst of an illness, injury, or major life change, so try practicing

> With time and practice, you will be able to ask in a calm, easy manner.

and preparing now. Use small opportunities to practice, learn, and grow in this area. If you do, it's likely that, like Marty and Olie in their stories below, you'll be ready if there's a need. Or, like Jeff, you'll at least be ready to begin thinking about it.

Marty's Letter to the Firm's Partners

Well everyone,

I shouldn't have believed you all when you said I was too mean to ever get sick. Just can't trust you—us—lawyers.

Your cards, flowers, and visits have been wonderful. Never thought I'd need a family, although I made a couple of stabs at marriage. Seems you all have become my family in the last twelve years since Molly and I ended it. With my life it was just a matter of time until I'd need some sort of safety net.

The doctors say my heart attack was a whopper, and I'll need more procedures to even regain 40 percent functioning.

My counselor says I need a care-share team, and he understands that there are a lot of friends and colleagues who care about me. (Little does he know that you all just put up with me.)

Anyway, with his help I am holding a meeting—noon, next Wednesday in the large conference room—to try to begin organizing the personal and professional help I'll need during the next few months.

Show up at your own risk. We're bringing great sandwiches from Zabar's. No commitment required. Brainstorming only.

Love you all, Marty

Olie's E-mail: Important Changes in My Life

Dear friends,

I am writing to inform you of an important change in my life. As some of you already know, a few weeks ago Collette and I separated. At the moment, we are working through the divorce process. For me, this has been a tough choice, but necessary for my future. Collette was hurt at first, but not completely surprised. During the past few weeks I've found that letting people know about this major change helps me quite a bit emotionally, so I thought I'd reach out with an e-mail, even to those friends who are physically far away. You may do whatever you want with this information.

What will happen in the short term? Right now, Collette and I are finalizing the divorce agreement. In all likelihood it will be another five to six months before everything is finalized. I want to reassure you that during this time Collette has complete access to health insurance through my employer, as well as exclusive use of our car and our condo in Bellevue. What will happen in the long term? I will let Collette tell you about her own plans for the future, if she chooses to do so, but for the next year and a half, I will be busy working and finishing my PhD. After that I will continue working as a researcher at the University of Washington.

What can you do? I don't need anything in particular from you, even though a phone call or an e-mail is always welcome. The only thing I ask is that those of you who are good friends with both Collette and me continue to be friends with both of us. I am doing very well. My parents have helped me enormously in these tough weeks, and I am now happily independent. Collette will probably need more help, not so much emotional, but practical. Because I don't want to presume to know her needs, I will let her express them to you, if she wants to.

Thanks for caring, Olie

Jeff's Waiting-Room Thoughts

Jeff was sitting in the lobby of a well-known cancer center, waiting for his appointment. Except for some minor surgeries, he had always been the healthy person and the one providing the help. This waiting room felt totally foreign to him.

He watched as one elderly gentleman carefully tended to his wheelchair-bound wife, while another nearby couple seemed worlds apart: Hubby was sitting a distance away from his wife, who sat blankly, a hat covering her hairless head. If Jeff hadn't seen the two of them enter the office together, he would have thought them strangers to each other.

"What would my experience be like?" he wondered. Would my family reject me or become distant? Would I share the intimacy of the first couple with my wife?" Then he remembered a book he had read years before, Counting on Kindness by Wendy Lustbader. He thought about many friends he had assisted on journeys into and through illness. He wondered how it would be now that he was the one facing cancer. He felt fortunate he hadn't had to ask for much help thus far in life. Slowly, it occurred to him that he would need to ask for help. He didn't know how to do it, but he came from a long line of survivors, and if help was needed he'd somehow ask for and get it.

FRIENDS AND RELATIVES RESPOND TO HELP APPEAL

If you have a friend who is feeling out of control and uncomfortable just asking for help—how will you respond? Instead of simply asking, "Is there anything I can do?" consider offering more: "Can you think of anything right now that I might do?" or "May I call you in the next few days to see how you're doing and to again ask how I might help?" or "If you think of anything I might do, or if you just want to talk, or if you just want to spend time together and not even talk about any of this, will you please pick up the phone, dial my number, and let me know?" Each of these offers leaves room for the person who seems to be in need to think about what might be helpful, to take control, and to give a more thoughtful reply.

In the following example, Steve calls back his friend Mark, who had left a message about his medical diagnosis.

> ### Steve's Voice-Mail Offer to Help
>
> Mark, we got your message on Sunday. I'm sorry I haven't called back sooner. It kind of hit me just like a punch in the stomach when you were describing the diagnosis. I felt a mixture of anger at the disease and love and care for you and Sylvi, but then I'm sure you're going through ten-fold beyond what I can imagine.
>
> But just wanted to let you know we got the message.

I've been thinking a lot about you and praying for your health, your good care, and good counsel from your medical advisors.

The most important thing to me right now is that once your treatment regimen becomes clear, I really hope I can be a part of that team that will hopefully help you defeat the disease. I really want to play a role for you, Mark, in that battle. Please know that we'll be there, whatever it takes.

Again, our thoughts and prayers are with you, Sylvi, and the boys.

Mariah is someone else who was surprised with a scary diagnosis. At age twenty-eight, her liver was dying. When this was diagnosed as a genetic disorder, primary sclerosing cholangitis, she and her husband, Tom, knew they had to look beyond family members for help. They established a Web site through www.caringbridge.com and used it to notify friends, former co-workers, and church members of the situation, to ask for help, and to keep all of them up to date. Here are some responses to Mariah's Web site.

E-mail Messages Responding to Mariah's Help Appeal

Dear Mariah,

I have been keeping up with you on your Web site. I just want you to know that I think of you often . . . and I am hoping you get out of the hospital soon. Please let me know if there is anything I can do to help with you or Jonah. Emily misses him; she does not understand why he is not in school with her. Please know that you are in my thoughts and prayers.

– Ann

Dear Mariah and Tom,

Let us know what we can do for you this weekend, if anything. If you need me to bring you home, I'll be happy to do so. If you need us to keep Jonah while Tom brings you home, we'll do that, too. I am happy to see your numbers coming down. Let's hope they stay there now that the duct is no longer blocked. I didn't call last night because I didn't want to wake you, but I'll try to call tonight.

Love, Dad

Hi Mariah,

I hope you are feeling better. I am so sorry to read that you had to go back to Georgetown again. Please let me now if there is anything I can do, especially now that Tom has gone back to work. I know you have neighbors, but I am not that far away. Michael, my older son, started school this past Monday and Sam starts preschool next week. Best of luck to Jonah on his first day of school. Michael started third grade this year, and I still cried when he got on the school bus. It is so hard to let go. My prayers are with you. You are such an inspiration to me.

> *Lots of love, Josephine*

Hi again Mariah,

> *My voice is a little odd (I saw my own ENT on Friday), but I can talk. So if you are bored don't hesitate to call. Hang in there. I hope the doctors come up with some kind of idea for kicking this resistant infection for good. Big hugs! You are always in my thoughts, and I'm rooting for Jonah to have a wonderful kindergarten orientation!*

> *Love, Patrice*

Mariah,

> *It has been a very long time since high school. I have been busy myself battling cancer, but prayer goes a long way. I have had you and your family in my thoughts since you have been sick. Never give up hope, stay strong. You will be in my prayers.*

> *– Yolanda*

From the above examples, it's clear that not everyone who is asked to help will actually want to or be able to follow through. If you're the one doing the asking it's important to not take this personally. Everyone in your circle has her own circumstances and personal history that will affect her capacity to say yes to your invitation. This was true for some of Mariah's family and friends, and also true for Charles. After a car accident, Charles asked for help for his wife, Mary, who had suffered dreadful injuries and expected a long recovery.

> Not everyone who is asked to help will actually want to or be able to follow through.

Jenny and Ray Respond

Hi Mary and Charles,

This is Jenny. Ray and I were so saddened to hear about the terrible car accident.

We pray for a rapid recovery for all five of you. We understand that Mary will need several surgeries, and we especially pray for her.

Ray and I would like to be a part of the care-share team you mentioned in your letter. My 93-year-old mom back in Atlanta, however, is sick, and Ray and I are going back to stay with her. We hope to convince her to move out here. As soon as we get back next week, we'll get in touch and help out. We'll pray for all of you. Bye for now.

Unlike Mariah and Tom, who liked using e-mail, some people, such as Glenn in the example below, prefer face-to-face interaction when bringing important news. Glenn took a very public risk, inviting fellow members of his Rotary group to help when he needed it.

Glenn's Invitation and the Response

"This is really serious," Glenn said, addressing his Rotary group. "This is really serious," he repeated. With voice faltering, he began, "I have just been diagnosed with pancreatic cancer and my odds aren't good. I joined this Rotary eight years ago to help others, and now I'm going to need help. I hope I'm not shocking you all too much, but you're my friends and I wanted you to know."

Following Glenn's moving help appeal, Howard, the former Rotary president, stood up and spoke. With heartfelt emotion, Howard expressed his concern for Glenn and that he knew he was speaking for all the men and women present: "We will be there for you. If there is anything we can do to help, however small or large, we want to know. You've given so much to others and we're happy to give back to you. Please keep us updated on your progress and your needs."

A few weeks later, a fellow Rotary member distributed copies of a form "What Can I Offer?" to each member to complete. Here is a sample segment of this form from our workbook.

WHAT CAN I OFFER?*

Name _Erika_

Address

Home Phone _206-123-4561_ Work Phone

Fax _____ Cell Phone _206-981-6543_

E-mail Address

AVAILABILITY

What are the best days and times for you to help?

Day/Time	Mon	Tues	Wed	Thurs	Fri	Sat	Sun
Morning							
Afternoon							
Evening				X			
Varies	X					X	X

FAMILY SUPPORT/CHILDREN
☐ Pick up car pool
☒ Child-focused attention
☐ Other: _____

MEALS
☒ Grocery shop
☐ Cook
☐ Assist with eating
☒ Wash dishes
☐ Share a meal
☐ Other: _____

TELEPHONE
☒ Telephone check-ins
☐ Medication reminder
☐ Special needs telephone
☐ Other: _____

FRIENDLY COMPANIONSHIP
☒ Personal shopping
☐ Social outing
☒ Hospital visit
☒ Talk/visit
☐ Other: _____

MEDICATIONS
☐ Remember
☐ Procure
☒ Coordinate
☐ Track
☐ Other: _____

* This is a sample portion of a form you may wish to create or that will be found in our workbooks.

The completed forms were given to Glenn, who expressed gratitude for this method of communicating caring words and concrete offers of help. In the following months, Glenn called upon his fellow Rotarians for help, ranging from driving him to and from chemotherapy infusions, to friendly companionship of eating pizza and watching a video, to running errands and buying groceries during the worst of Glenn's fatigue.

GET READY

Ask yourself:	If I were to write a help-appeal letter or script, how would it begin? (Try a few times to really do this.)
Think:	Can I take no for an answer without being crushed or angry? Am I grateful when I receive help?
Be honest:	Do I like to help others? Have I been able to say yes and no to past requests for help?
Decide:	If I need to ask for help, will I prefer to phone, write, meet, or e-mail?
Count:	How many times have I actually used this method? Do I need help to begin?

CHAPTER 4
Take the First Steps

Now that you've joined or formed a care-share team to assist a care partner—to help her live a fuller and healthier life while confronting one of life's surprises—what happens next? Care teams really need to focus on the care partner: What does she want? What needs does she have that aren't being met? How can her life be enhanced?

Toward this end, you will convene with a variety of people, asking questions and volunteering time, talents, and energy to ease the care partner's isolation and difficulties. There are some basic, logical steps you can take to effectively coordinate these efforts: Appoint a leader, schedule regular meetings, establish ground rules, state your shared values, figure out what's needed, and make a plan for meeting those needs. All the while, you'll want to keep your care partner's needs as the primary focus.

> Keep your care partner's needs as the primary focus.

Staying focused on your care partner's needs is also going to require you to sometimes give up control. One team member's way of doing things may not be the way the care partner prefers. Within reason, respecting and honoring the care partner's right to self-determination and self-control is important for her well-being and emotional health.

One way to begin is to assist your care partner in defining her needs. The sample form below is a starting point; we include an expanded form in our workbook.

WHAT MIGHT BE NEEDED?*

Name *Paul*
(person for whom care-share team is being designed)

Date *July 21, 2006*

HEALTH/PERSONAL CARE
- ☒ Exercise/walking
- ☐ Blood pressure
- ☐ Nail care
- ☐ Haircuts/shampoos
- ☐ Massages
- ☐ Other: _____

FINANCIAL
- ☒ Sort bills
- ☒ Balance bank statement
- ☐ Insurance papers
- ☐ Pay bills
- ☐ Other: _____

HOUSEHOLD CHORES
- ☒ Vacuum/dust
- ☐ Wash floor/windows
- ☐ Clean refrigerator
- ☐ Remove trash
- ☒ Laundry
- ☐ Other: _____

PET/PLANT CARE
- ☒ Feed/exercise pets
- ☒ Water/trim plants
- ☐ Other: _____

YARD/GARDEN WORK
- ☒ Mow/trim/rake
- ☐ Shovel snow
- ☒ Tend to flower garden
- ☐ Clean gutters
- ☐ Other: _____

READING/WRITING
- ☐ Record life stories
- ☐ Read books/newspapers
- ☒ Write letters/cards
- ☐ Help sort mail

HOME REPAIRS
- ☒ Paint
- ☐ Simple carpentry
- ☐ Repairs
- ☐ Light home maintenance
- ☐ Install grab bars/railings
- ☐ Other: _____

TRANSPORTATION
- ☐ Medical appointments
- ☒ Shopping/errands
- ☐ Car maintenance

* This is a sample portion of a form you may wish to create or that will be found in our workbooks.

In the first story below, the care receiver, Ann, was cooperative and capable of enlisting aid from others. In the second story, family dynamics made it difficult for anyone to step in to help.

Ann's Story

When Ann became ill enough that she and her husband alone couldn't handle all of the details of life, some of us who were close to her and part of her informal safety net formed a team, consisting of a paid caregiver, a therapist interested in group dynamics and aging, one family member, a case manager, neighbors, and some of her friends and former colleagues. These folks gathered to see how they might help Ann live the life she envisioned for herself. Ann listed what she needed help with: grocery shopping, companionship, sending cards and letters, bill paying, cooking, outings, and accompanying her to doctor's appointments. Those present clarified what time and interests they could contribute.

Even if there's a clear picture of what's needed, it will still be important for one person to take a lead role. Even in dire situations, such as the one in the following story, strong leadership can succeed.

A Strong Professional Team Leader Was Required

The *oldest son phoned me, explaining that the family had just fired the second social worker, after having fired a nurse care manager, all three of whom had attempted to coordinate the care of this family's ninety-two-year-old mother. Her fragility, unsteadiness on her feet, and inability to care for herself due to "memory lapses"—combined with a fierce independence— made care coordination important, though family dynamics presented challenges. The son added, "I fired the last social worker because she couldn't keep peace among us, and she wouldn't make some of us do what we said we were going to do. I want you to know this history. If you can't do better, then we don't need to talk and waste our time." A strong leader was needed to maintain peace* among a strong-willed, very loyal, and often at-odds group of three brothers, two sisters, two involved daughters-in-law, and two granddaughters.

In this situation, a paid professional was invited to try to bring cooperation and teamwork out of disagreements, anger, and disorganization. The family's loyalty to this beloved woman was clear. To transform this fierce safety net, however, into a well-functioning team, strong leadership was required. Through both of the stories above, you can see that selecting a leader is a logical first step.

APPOINT A LEADER

Soon after you've established a care-share team, you will want to select one person to take the lead. The care partner, if capable and willing, could possibly step into this role, as Ann did. Or perhaps a spouse, child, sibling, or friend can. Some groups hire a professional counselor (as in the case of the family in the story above). Whether this person volunteers, is nominated, or is hired by the group, this leader or coordinator often writes up a schedule; acts as the point or hub person for conflicts; and sets a date, time, and location for a first gathering. He can make the contacts and set the agenda or delegate some of these tasks. Then, when the team meets, this leader may also act as facilitator who will keep the meeting focused and solicit input from everyone (though another person with tact and skill in this area may want to handle this task). He may take and distribute meeting notes that clearly define commitments of who will do what, and when. Additionally, he will continually

> Choosing a leader—other than the care partner—is a way of lightening his or her burden, not layering on tasks.

update the schedule and roster or delegate these tasks to someone who is good at paying attention to detail.

Choosing a leader—other than the care partner—is a way of lightening his or her burden, not layering on tasks. Some leaders go to great lengths to ease another's burden. Look at the example in the fictionalized story below.

Susan Stewart

Susan Stewart has come back from Iraq, though not to the homecoming she and her family had envisioned. While on patrol duty, Susan was seriously injured when her vehicle was hit. A fellow soldier was killed. Risking their own safety, other soldiers pulled Susan from the wreckage, into a safe area, and toward emergency medical treatment. Infections and complications set in, forcing Susan to return to her hometown Veterans Administration hospital for recovery and rehabilitation.

While in the hospital, Susan met a caring volunteer who offered to work with Susan's family and local townspeople to create a team to help Susan through the hard times ahead. Together they faced Susan's complex and challenging new realities. This veteran volunteer provided strong leadership for the many members—young and old—who stepped up to the plate and formed Susan's care team. Volunteers helped remodel Susan's parents' home to accommodate Susan's wheelchair. Church members hosted an old-fashioned ice-cream social to raise money. Health-care providers offered outpatient services at no or very low cost to Susan. Best of all, *the volunteers didn't view this as a hardship: It seemed a fitting way to say thank you for the sacrifice Susan had made to help protect her country. And it started with the willingness, vision, and leadership of one hospital volunteer—and a wider safety net to keep it going.*

Though most team leaders probably can't go to such incredible lengths, Susan Stewart's story illustrates the power of an effective leader believing the community could be a safety net and organizing a supportive team around someone who needs help.

PLAN THE FIRST MEETING

After you've chosen a leader and set a meeting time, you will plan the first meeting. Ideally at the first meeting you will make introductions, ask each person why he or she has come, define the group's vision (read more about that below), and begin to formulate a care plan and a schedule.

This is the time to get ideas and opinions flowing, and decide who's in and who will do what for an initial period of time. Begin by identifying the five or ten most important tasks, instead of tackling everything all at once. When you jump ahead without a plan, even though well-intentioned, you may easily end up feeling like you're spinning your wheels. Start out on the right foot by creating a care plan and breaking down this plan into a list of manageable tasks. Write down specifics and post them. Then ask each person to select one task from this list. Encourage each person to start small and then expand his role. (This works better than promising too much upfront, then having to cut back later.) After a while, people who've become comfortable being around the care partner might add more time or tasks; others may cut back or drop out altogether.

> Encourage each person to start small and then expand his role. (This works better than promising too much upfront, then having to cut back later.)

The idea is to set a working vision and move forward. Set a schedule and encourage everyone to stick to it. But be realistic: Plan for the unexpected. Figure out ahead of time what'll happen if someone can't handle what they're scheduled to do. Being sick, having a car break down, or leaving town for a last-minute business trip can play havoc with the best-crafted schedule. It's best if a team member who cannot do what has been planned takes responsibility for finding a replacement or contacting the coordinator. Communicate with your team. Use tools, such as a phone tree or an e-mail group list, to find a substitute. Assign a scheduler (either the team leader or someone she delegates this assignment to) who is the hub for such times and who keeps a list of potential short notice fill-ins.

What time should the schedule cover? A week is too short. A year is often too long. Probably, at least in the beginning, a month or quarter is about right. The following sample calendar has been adapted from our companion workbook. Feel free to use these ideas as you create your schedule.

CALENDAR*

MONTH

Sun	Mon	Tues	Wed	Thurs	Fri	Sat
	1	2	3	4	5	6
	10am-noon Mary pool	1-2:30pm Tom sit and talk 4pm Susan to MD		10am-noon Mary pool		5:30pm Lil for dinner

CST MEMBERS   WORK PHONE   HOME PHONE   E-MAIL

Susan _____

Tom _____

Danny _____

Lil _____

Mary _____

EMERGENCY NUMBERS FOR CARE PARTNER

Main Doctor _____

Power of Attorney _____

Durable Health _____

Family Member _____

Insurance _____

MEDICAL INFORMATION FOR CARE PARTNER

Name and Address _____

Social Security _____

Birth Date _____

Blood Type _____

Allergies _____

Medications _____

* This is a sample portion of a form you may wish to create or that will be found in our workbooks.

After setting a schedule, your next priority is meeting together regularly. This gives you all an opportunity to mention outstanding needs, gain information, support each other when the task becomes difficult, and provide for the emotional well-being of members who may be frightened, challenged, or angered by some aspect of the caregiving role. You can also express appreciation for one another's contributions, celebrate

> It's important to guard one another's privacy and keep details from spreading to a broader circle.

successes, and enjoy coming together for a common purpose. What's more, face-to-face meetings allow you to address needs and concerns. If these are too big for the team to handle, this may be where an adept individual or a professional is called.

ESTABLISH SOME GROUND RULES

At the outset, as well as when your team takes shape and begins to function, establish some ground rules. Here are a few common rules that many teams use:

1. Maintain confidentiality. Keep the sensitive information gathered in a meeting inside the team. Avoid gossip: This includes anything from health or scheduling data to clarifying whether or not your care partner wants to reveal

the nature of an existing issue. It definitely includes avoiding gossip about what's going on in the lives of other team members. You and your team will likely become close to and supportive of each other, but it's important to guard one another's privacy and keep details from spreading to a broader circle.

2. Set limits on your availability: Do not take on a task you're uncomfortable with or commit to more time than you can really give. Offer only what you can actually accomplish. No one knows for sure how long a care team will exist; it's easier to avoid burnout than to deal with it later. Learning early to only offer what you can, to set limits, is valuable, as is building in opportunities to revise schedules and tasks as you go. This is part of why a team has the potential to work better for longer than a buddy or familial set up. There are more hands and heads to lend to the tasks. Working as a team allows all of you to take well-earned breaks and tend to the other important parts of your lives.

3. Be on time. Starting and ending meetings on time is respectful of all parties. Try hard to keep them short. Show the same consideration to your care partner, who may be leading a life filled with limitations on mobility. Waiting for an anticipated visit becomes an important part of the day. Being late can raise anxiety for the care partner—certainly not anyone's goal.

4. Keep purse strings tight. It is easy to complicate a relationship with loans or cash gifts. Treats of an occasional cup of coffee or cookies for a meeting are fine, but paying for a doctor's visit, or renting a wheelchair, can easily grow into either dependency or resentment. It's far better for a team to brainstorm ideas on how to take care of a need.

> Creating rituals to honor an important transition often helps all concerned recognize and deal with the change.

Contacting a social service agency may be appropriate in figuring out how to provide items or services. The team itself is not a social service agency, but it does pull together the resources to contact and work with one or several. We have repeatedly seen how gifts of money can complicate things more than anticipated.

5. Show respect. As a team, take the time to compile a list of behaviors that show respect for one another. Post this list to help ease tense moments. Avoid "cross-talk," which is shifting the focus of conversation away from the work of the care-share team and toward yourself. Interrupting, likewise, is most often disrespectful. Help each other avoid such behaviors.

6. Honor endings. Endings inevitably come, whether it's a timely end to a meeting, the departure of a team member, the death of the care partner, or the physical recovery of the care partner. Creating rituals to honor an important transition often helps all concerned recognize and deal with the change. (Read more about this in the Keep Rituals and Traditions section of Chapter 5.)

My Grandparents' Story

Every night at 5:30 p.m., Grandpa would be pushed in his wheelchair into the room where Gram was reclining on the couch. "My dear, you look lovely tonight." he'd say, "Would you like to join me for a cocktail?" She'd reply, "Oh, Walter, I'm so glad to see you. I'd love a Manhattan." And Grandpa would turn to the person propelling his chair to ask that drinks be served.

Neither of my grandparents could walk independently, yet those around them created the space and provided the "legs" for their nightly ritual, so important to both of them. My grandparents were still in charge of their own lives, and their care-share team worked to safeguard that independence. Maintaining small habits, routines, or rituals can play a critical role in protecting the quality of life for vulnerable and ill people when so much else may be changing, uncertain, or lost. There is a delicate and ever-changing balance.

CLARIFY VISION AND VALUES

Two of the most important tasks a newly formed team can do are to define a group vision and to compile a group list of values. Ask yourselves, "Why are we helping? What do we hope to make happen?" When you put these answers into a brief vision statement and a list of values, you'll create a road map to follow as you participate in this new community. Frequently remind

> "Why are we helping? What do we hope to make happen?"

the team about the shared vision and values that have brought you all together. When you're faced with ambiguous decisions and situations, these provide focus and glue. A team's vision statement may be as simple as "We will support Dan and Corie during this difficult pregnancy," as was true for the team in the next story. Try to state an active vision. Avoid having it be tied to one specific outcome, since none of us can see the future. A general vision statement tied to a hope-filled outcome allows for variation. Values will evolve from this.

Dan and Corie's Values

Dan and Corie invited family, friends, and neighbors into a care *team when Corie was bedridden during the second month of her pregnancy. After three months, it became clear that crisis was following crisis. To Dan, it seemed Corie was part of the problem: She wasn't following the doctor's orders or accepting help. And the team was wearing down. At a scheduled care-share meeting, Dan brought up the issue, asking members to share feelings and brainstorm ideas to break out of the cycle. Together, the team restated the value of holding continuing connection with friends and relatives. They reaffirmed their desire to hold curiosity and compassion when faced with problems like this one. They reassured Corie that the team existed for her benefit,* and that having a difficulty was not a bad thing, but could lead to creative solutions and positive outcomes.

When the team expressed their frustration, Corie could then understand how her actions affected the people she loved—and needed—most. Once Corie accepted her temporary dependence on others, she could begin thinking creatively about community and connection. In the next story, Trisha's team relied on their four stated values when it came time to make choices that were in the best interest of their care partner.

Trisha's Move

In our care-share team, when we need to reach a decision or prioritize, we use a set of four values that have emerged over time: safety, security, serenity, and simplicity. The alliteration helps us remember them. When we are discussing something in our care partner's life and are having difficulty reaching a decision, remembering these values helps us set priorities.

For instance, when Trisha was given the chance to change rooms in the facility where she lives, we talked about her options with an eye toward safety: Would the new room be more or less safe than the current one? We talked about her feelings of security and serenity: Where did she feel most able to be herself and sink down roots? We talked about simplicity: What about the new space would contribute to living simply? Trisha then made a decision based on these values and priorities. She admitted that, without a team, she'd have skipped this process. She loved the result.

Trisha decided to move, but she waited until an appropriate first-floor room was vacant. She talked with the management about the details of the move so that team members would not have to supply the labor. She honored her needs for more light and air in the new space while paying attention to keeping the move organized, purposeful, and *positive.*

With this well-thought-out decision, team members felt assured that their friend's inclination toward spontaneity and self-expression wouldn't lead to crises and chaos. They embraced the move and each lent a hand to make the new room a home—when it was time.

MANAGE CHOICES AND DECISIONS

You and the other care team members may not agree with all of your care partner's, or her surrogate decision maker's, choices. This can pose a dilemma.

For example, if a care partner elects to have a surgery that entails a high level of risk and a low chance for success, it might be difficult for you to affirm this choice. You may fear that this will create an even greater crisis and a higher level of need. You might feel torn between wanting to protect the care partner's right to make her own decisions and your own right to limit what you offer her.

> You might feel torn between wanting to protect the care partner's right to make her own decisions and your own right to limit what you offer her.

At other times, a care partner may continue to engage in risky behavior, while still asking

for help. While refocusing on the shared vision and values may frequently help resolve such dilemmas, others may involve competing values and prove more difficult. At that point, you will need to reflect deeply upon your reasons for choosing to be supportive. It's equally important for the care partner to show sensitivity and respect toward you and the other team members. As much as possible, keep an open dialogue and perhaps seek professional facilitation to define roles, limits, and areas of compromise. And remember, circumstances change: Not everyone will be well-suited to participate for the full life of the care-share team.

Saying No to Grandma

When my grandmother became incapacitated, her sleep habits changed. Somehow her mixed-up body perked up at night and rested only during daytime hours. When she called on us to help her in the middle of the night, we began humoring her, comparing her to Henry Kissinger, who reputedly conducted meetings in foreign countries on his Washington, D.C. timetable. After a while, however, we acknowledged that we hadn't taken care of ourselves. We had to give Grandmother a "curfew" and impose limits on our availability. While Grandma definitely disliked this change, it caused no irreparable damage and helped us better manage our own lives.

Your challenge may become holding the care partner's needs, preferences, and values as primary but also considering your needs and those of the care team. Balancing needs is a complex task requiring self-knowledge, communication skills, and flexibility. In many situations, outside professionals may help by facilitating discussions when there are tensions between hopes, fears, preferences, values, and objectives.

Most times, the care partner will identify his own needs and the way in which they are met. In other cases the care partner and a trusted loved one, or the team as a whole, will collaborate to define needs and ways to meet those needs. In still other cases, such as advanced mental deterioration (for example, the late stages of Alzheimer's disease), someone other than the care partner must handle these decisions. In all cases, you should keep values and lifestyle in mind when making decisions for him.

Appointing a Health Care Power of Attorney is an important part of planning.

When a care partner is legally deemed no longer able to make sound judgments but had the foresight to legally specify a Health Care Power of Attorney to make health-care decisions, then that person can speak on his behalf. In the unfortunate case where no appointment was made, then someone will be appointed—but this may not be someone the care partner would select. Appointing a Health Care Power of Attorney is an important part of planning.

Balancing needs becomes even more complex when the care partner is a child or when the team is supporting the entire family. Obviously, a child's welfare and well-being is dependent upon his parents, who, in turn, rely heavily on their own safety net. Therefore the care-share team most often supports the needs of the whole family. The following story of Crystal is an example of this working well.

Crystal's Cystic Fibrosis

Eight-year-old Crystal and her entire family were challenged and forever changed by her cystic fibrosis. Crystal's mom, Elaine, relied on her own best friend, Elizabeth, from the start. Elizabeth, in turn, recruited, encouraged, and guided many of their mutual friends into various helping roles. Because their kids went to the same school and they attended the same church, Elizabeth had ample opportunity to support and guide the actions of this loosely defined team.

Elizabeth often invited Elaine's sons, who were the same age as her two sons, for sleepovers during Crystal's many hospital stays. During her long transplant, Crystal's two brothers were well taken care of as many other parents shared in car-pooling, sporting events, and sleepovers. Because Elizabeth rallied other families to pitch in, the family's trauma was lessened and life went on despite the heartache of Crystal's final and difficult year of life.

No matter the age of the person you're helping, offer your support in a manner consistent with her needs, values, and preferences (or of those speaking for her). Author Mary Oliver reminds us that "playfulness, grace and humor, those inseparable spirits of vitality" are invaluable. Using gentleness of phrase, humor to maintain a sense of balance, and opportunities for playfulness will serve everyone well. And as you go about your work, remember these three basic assumptions: Keep the care partner at the center of the care-share team; do only what you can freely offer; and speak up respectfully, especially when anything uncomfortable comes up.

> Using gentleness of phrase, humor to maintain a sense of balance, and opportunities for playfulness will serve everyone well.

HANDLE THE COMPLEXITIES OF MONEY

In most safety net scenarios, people's access to and relationship with money varies widely. It's simplest to not spend your own money on the care partner's expenses. When you do, expectations of continued spending, reactions or jealousies by other team members, loans mistaken for gifts, secrecy, and a host of other dilemmas crop up. A precedent might be set that can become increasingly uncomfortable and hard to address. On the other hand, each situation is unique. Some team members may have an established history of gift giving or spending their own money on the care partner. Before you give of your own resources, be aware of the potential complexity of the exchange of money. Then, discuss with the whole team your wishes in handling this issue. Use team meeting time to address financial matters head on: Together, you and the group can reach clear and sustainable solutions.

> Together, you and the group can reach clear and sustainable solutions.

More about Martha

As the disease progressed, so did Martha's money woes. Without her health, there just wasn't a way for Martha to stay employed. It seemed unfair that she'd lose her apartment and her health insurance. Despite her attempts to keep her helpers apart, over time some of them met each other and eventually discussed some of the more complicated issues.

Money was one of these issues. At the time of her final hospitalization, the team made the realistic decision to relinquish Martha's apartment and put everything in storage. They then contacted Martha' family members, pooled their resources to pay for one month of storage space, and boxed up Martha's belongings for storage until a family member could come and make final arrangements.

You may be tempted to see yourself as the "saving angel," but stepping into this role takes important identity away from the care partner as well as decreases both the buy-in and the scope of other care-share team members. As you walk through this journey with your care partner and team, sensitivity about financial issues may be an ongoing challenge and lesson. We both have learned many lessons the hard way and will no doubt learn more.

> You can help simplify your care partner's life, and lower his expenses, when you know the full picture of all the prescriptions he is taking.

REVIEW MEDICATIONS

It is not our intent to try to give specific advice on medications. What's important is that one person—ideally the team leader—periodically review *all* of

the care partner's medications with *one* physician. Medications can multiply as a person consults with different specialists, and it's wise to designate one physician who will act as the switchboard operator. What's more, interactions between medicines can generate surprising results. Some puzzling behaviors can be the result of drug interactions. You can help simplify your care partner's life, and lower his expenses, when you know the full picture of all the prescriptions he is taking. Keep a log of what medicine was prescribed by which physician and when. This will prove to be a helpful tool when a physician needs to reevaluate a medication or in case of a health crisis.

This is another situation where you'll need to balance the care partner's privacy with your ability to provide appropriate care. Carefully weigh each unique situation: Let your care partner's level of comfort with transparency and openness guide your decisions.

FIGURE OUT WHAT'S NEEDED

Whenever you take part in a care team, you'll discover that there are some rather standard tasks, and others that are highly personalized. No matter the situation—illness, injury, frailty, divorce, birth of a child, time of grieving, or end of life—you can tailor your response to the unique need.

It's good to maintain an open mind and heart about what is possible. Brainstorming needs, listing skills and availabilities, seeing where there are gaps, and doing more brainstorming about ways to fill these are all good early steps. Maybe your group can't fill every need: That's when some prioritizing needs to happen. As in the earlier story of Hugh and Megan, there may be a long list of needs. Hugh decided to extend his team by hiring some help and using friends and family for the things they were best at. If money had been an issue, he might have researched other avenues or invited other people in. He was fortunate to have a large safety net from which the smaller care-share team originated. Or, some needs might have gone unmet, leading to more prioritizing.

Will's Prostate Cancer: Ken as Team Leader

Men can be hardheaded and stubborn, and want to keep illnesses, surgeries, and health conditions to themselves. Will was an exception. He worked in the high-tech industry, where forming and reforming teams to accomplish objectives and create products was the norm. When he was diagnosed with prostate cancer, he recognized immediately that his wife, who worked and carried the bulk of the responsibilities for their nine-year-old daughter and eleven-year-old son, would not be able to provide all of the help he would need. Nor did Will think she should. He adored his wife and respected the way she balanced parenting and directing the marketing department of a small firm. He wanted to protect her so she could continue these things. He was also realistic about what his needs and limitations might be.

Will's creating a care-share team was propelled along by his conversation with his best friend and work colleague, Ken. During a long lunch when Will shared his news, Ken assured him, "Well, count me in. I want to know all the details, and to be a key player in this team. We'll see you through this illness and out the other side. I'll be there for you until this project is successfully accomplished, too."

After some private thinking and discussions with his wife, Will followed his wife's suggestion and asked Ken not only to be a part of the team but also to lead it. Ken was touched by the trust his friend placed in him. He agreed, but said he'd have to process it in his own fashion to "operationalize" project goals as he phrased it before they could form a team. The others willingly followed his lead.

Thus began one very successful care-share team in which Ken played an important lead role in supporting his friend Will. Ken used his valuable tech project management experience to quietly, efficiently, and sensitively build and maintain a team "project" that saw Will and his family through many difficult days.

Remembering the care partner's unique needs, as well as each team member's gifts, is essential for creating the best care team. Regardless of how good the planning is, however, it's also valuable to keep a sense of humor nearby. Humor can diffuse or soften many potentially difficult situations, as can prayer, if that's something that's part of the team culture.

Tori's Challenge: John's Humor

There was a lot of humor in my first meeting with Tori, a powerful, independent, smart care partner who was angry because her disease brought a premature end to her accomplished career. While still beautiful in most people's eyes, Tori was very sensitive to the disease having taken one eye, which forced her to wear what she thought was a very noticeable artificial eye. She was sensitive about people's reactions to her prosthetic eye. I was interviewing her, and she was interviewing me, to see if I would become a paid counselor for her and a professional member of her team. During the interview, Tori suddenly reached up, popped out her artificial eye, and handed it to me. With strong, if quaking, nerves I replied, "Oh, you want to see if we can see eye to eye." She sighed, laughed, put the eye back in, and said that I "might just last."

Clearly, there will be times of tension when needs can't be met or when people may not get along easily. In addition to praying, prioritizing, and keeping a sense of humor, remembering that this is a time- and task-limited sort of family may help. It's not likely to last forever. Also, remember that the goal here is to be helpful, and to do so in a way that respects all participants.

You may not have the luxury or the control to hand pick and retain the ideal team from an unlimited number of friends, neighbors, relatives, paid social and health-care professionals, and others who volunteer to comprise your personal safety net. Therefore, you must be practical and creative. Expect that your team will evolve, sometimes based on the needs of the person receiving care, sometimes based on the needs of people giving care, and sometimes on the fickle finger of fate.

Ed's Care-Share Team Keeps Growing

When Ed suffered a heart attack, his wife, Elita, sent out an e-mail to family and close friends. As time passed and Ed had extensive tests and quadruple by-pass surgery, he, or Elita, would talk with other friends, colleagues, or church members about Ed's condition. People usually were interested and asked if there was anything they could do. Elita and Ed would thank them and tell them of the e-mail report, the "Ed Report" as Elita called it, and ask if they would like to be added to the list. Soon the list grew to forty-three people. Not everyone on the list lived close by, so they contributed by praying, calling, and sending notes of encouragement. Some who lived in town provided transportation, meals, and help with household chores, which allowed Elita to take time off during the long months of Ed's recovery.

It's been said that "life is 10 percent what happens to you and 90 percent what you do with it." Once you're in a care-share situation, it's important to make your best efforts to meet needs head on.

The care-share relationship is dynamic and changing. You will be looking for ideas, and sometimes these fresh ideas come from people who approach things differently than you do. A person who is difficult—who never goes with the majority—may want to join the team. Though this can present challenges, it's not necessarily a negative. Inviting this "stranger" into the midst of your team can provide a useful contrast to the group opinion and perhaps provide different ideas and skills. At times, in fact, the "stranger" is exactly who is needed. This may be the ex-spouse, the youth in a group of adults, the Muslim in a mostly Buddhist group—in other words, the unexpected. In *Gracious Space*, Pat Hughes notes this:

> **Sometimes these fresh ideas come from people who approach things differently than you do.**

"Community is dependent upon our willingness to invite the stranger . . . a true community is where we encounter people different from ourselves . . . a stranger is someone who thinks differently, acts differently or has a different background. . . . It is as if we each hold a piece of the puzzle. In order to complete the puzzle and resolve the issue, everyone needs to bring his or her piece. Not only will diverse perspectives help complete the puzzle, they can generate a breakthrough situation—one where a creative solution emerges from sharing different ideas. The greater the difference in thinking, the more creative the solution will likely be . . . in nature, diversity is insurance for life."

As you take your journey into caring, you—and the rest of the team—will inevitably face challenges. You will wish at times you were all like-minded—that would be the easiest course, especially in difficult scenarios. But this is exactly when the most creativity will be needed. Think twice before barring the door to strangers. As Pat Hughes so wisely reminds us, "Seeing the stranger as an ally, rather than an enemy, is central to dealing with complexity." Sometimes a way to gain this outside perspective is to add paid professionals to your safety net or care-share team. This can make a critical difference.

> As you take your journey into caring, you—and the rest of the team—will inevitably face challenges.

Floyd's Story

Floyd was an eighty-three-year-old legally blind man who called me at the advice of his accountant with whom he had worked for the past thirty-six years. Floyd had one son and one daughter, both of whom had busy professional lives and families on the opposite coast. Floyd, a highly successful business man, had become increasingly isolated following the death of his wife five years earlier and the deaths of several long-time friends. Floyd remained remarkably independent, living in his condominium within short walking distance of his bank, grocery store, dentist, and short taxi ride to his physician. However, his accountant, with whom Floyd usually met two or three times a year, could see that Floyd was becoming increasingly frail and therefore vulnerable to an accident or illness. He worried that no one would immediately notice and summon the medical attention Floyd needed.

Floyd's caring accountant laid out this concern to the family and offered some options. Floyd listened, but was resistant to this idea that was at odds with his accustomed independence. Recognizing that his poor eyesight did make him vulnerable to falls and because he preferred to pay someone, rather than ask his busy kids, Floyd hired a life-coach counselor to help set up a care-share team.

Here is how Floyd's team operated. First, Floyd and I, his counselor and life coach, created a list of people with phone numbers and e-mail addresses. Secondly, we wrote a letter and sent it to this proposed care team. The letter expressed appreciation and described our belief that the members needed to know how to reach each other in the event of an emergency. Floyd acknowledged that he was becoming frail and that he welcomed everyone to help him look out for himself.

GET READY

Ask yourself:	What unique skills can I contribute to this team? How much time can I commit on a regular basis?
Make a list:	Who would make an effective leader for this team? Should we hire a paid professional?
Make another list:	Jot down immediate needs in order of priority. Which tasks can I handle? Which responsibilities can I delegate?
Prepare:	Can I say no if someone asks for more time, energy, or money than I can freely give?

CHAPTER 5
Keep the Team Going

Joining a care-share team will bring both rewards and challenges to your life. People who have been part of teams speak often, and with passion, about the rewards they experience: a sense of connection, a greater awareness of the gift and fragility of life, and new wisdom gained from working with others. Being a part of someone's safety net in this way can be tremendously rewarding.

> At times helping won't feel good—because of time pressures, a cranky care partner, personal business that's being put off, and many other reasons.

But, realistically, at times helping won't feel good—because of time pressures, a cranky care partner, personal business that's being put off, and many other reasons. You may feel others are making unreasonable demands of you. You may feel guilty about not being able to accomplish everything. You may feel negative even when the care partner expresses gratitude for your help. For most people, though, these negatives pale in comparison to the positives. In fact, Multifaith Works, a Seattle nonprofit that invites people to join interfaith

care-share teams to support community members with HIV/AIDS or multiple sclerosis, has more volunteers than it can train. The word has spread that caring for others feels good.

In our years of caregiving, we've discovered simple strategies to maintain this goodwill within a group.

SCHEDULE ONGOING MEETINGS

Schedule regular check-in meetings. Encourage members to share experiences, concerns, and schedule conflicts. Many care-share teams reduce problems by routinely discussing how to cut back, take a break, or switch to less demanding tasks. Regularly scheduled meetings provide a forum where team members can ask for help if they're feeling overwhelmed. Sometimes professionals come in to train volunteers in specific aspects of the work.

Participating in a group where it's okay to speak of burnout, change, or cutting back creates a positive experience for everyone. It's only human to occasionally feel overwhelmed or tired; in the care-share team these feelings can be countered with information and, perhaps, training. Such feelings are normal, expected, and can be aired in a safe, supportive context. Regular meetings can function as a safety valve. This is the place where folks can speak of all the feelings that arise out of participation,

find compassionate listeners, and adjust roles and responsibilities.

Sticking to a set meeting schedule eliminates the need to repeatedly work out a new one. Once a month or once every other month is probably enough to keep things flowing, although some teams, especially during very difficult or intense times, may need to meet weekly. At each meeting, your group will want to accomplish the following:

- Check in with each other regarding events, emotions, or commitments that will affect the ability to be part of the team.
- Update the care partner's needs or schedule. Prioritize tasks if there are too many needs
- or wishes for the team to fulfill.
- Adjust the schedule to address ongoing or newly identified needs. Delete

> Regular meetings can function as a safety valve. This is the place where folks can speak of all the feelings that arise out of participation, find compassionate listeners, and adjust roles and responsibilities.

tasks that are no longer needed.

- Share pertinent information about the care partner. Keep in mind: This is not a gossip session, but rather an opportunity to learn what it will take to do a better and more compassionate job of support.

- Celebrate successes; have fun and play together to build cohesiveness and camaraderie.

If you participate in a care-share group that also includes the care partner, you will sometimes want to meet without him in order to freely air feelings that might hurt or offend. You can handle this in a straightforward way, reminding the team about the need to care for his heart. Team members must do their best to be honest but tactful with themselves and their team.

At times, though, it's helpful for the care partner to attend the team meetings. In the story below, a care-team member describes how involving her care partner in meetings and decisions benefited the whole team.

CARE PARTNER AS CARE-TEAM MEMBER

Although it is probably somewhat unusual to have the care partner as a regular member of the team, we include her in our team. Occasionally we've met without her, but I can't imagine how we'd have gone forward without the input of our care partner, who has a life-threatening progressive and episodic genetic disease. Over the years she's brought up not only issues for us to brainstorm but also terrific resolutions. Only she knows how she'll feel, and having her present allows her to share these feelings. However, there are also disadvantages, which we've worked around. Her medications have made her loopy or suspicious at times. This can be difficult or funny, but sometimes results in feedback about the side effects of medication to relay to the doctors. Overall, we've found

> You must use sensitivity and make decisions on a case-by-case basis, inevitably through some trial and error.

that engaging our care partner in our regular meetings works well because she gives us her direct input so we can discuss options in the moment.

As a general rule of thumb, however, the care partner does not always participate in the team meetings. She may be too ill, young, tired, stressed, or compromised to take part. In fact, you can think of the situation as similar to holding an executive board session. Your team may be talking about feelings, scheduling challenges, or group dynamics that are solvable, but may present an unnecessary burden and anxiety for the care partner. You must use sensitivity and make decisions on a case-by-case basis, inevitably through some trial and error.

COMMUNICATE

Frequent communication is as important as regularly scheduled meetings for team cohesion and team performance. Good communication begins with the team leader, who can take meeting notes, send them to everyone on the team, and use the notes as a tool for keeping everyone working together. The team leader also can regularly update schedules to maintain team member involvement and keep the information fresh. Even the smallest gestures can build team cohesion, such as asking everyone to pitch in to a collection kitty to cover the cost of stamps, paper, and envelopes.

> Be careful to communicate openly, not selectively, to avoid having some team members feel left out.

Be careful to communicate openly, not selectively, to avoid having some team members feel left out. A care partner's issues can trigger a team member's memories or fears. Everyone's feelings can be pretty raw when the care partner is going through a crisis or dealing with the pain and fear of a terrible illness, loss, or injury. Feelings can be easily bruised or hurt, so find ways to let every member know what's going on and that they are important. It is everybody's job to support each other.

Besides meeting notes, other useful tools are a phone tree and a group e-mail list. If you've had school-age children, you're probably familiar with the phone-tree way of relaying information from one person to another. Here is how it works: The care partner (or team leader) phones one person with information regarding a crisis or concern. This person then calls two or three others, each of whom then calls two or three more. If someone does not answer the phone, then an additional call needs to be made to the next person on the list until a voice-to-voice contact is made. Action may be needed, so it's crucial to take this step. Depending on the sensitivity of the information, messages can be left. Obviously, it's important for everyone listed on the phone tree to have an up-to-date copy of it. Here's an example:

PHONE TREE*

If you must send out information quickly, call the first person on the tree. The first person, in turn, must make contact directly with someone next on the list. Call until you reach someone, then go back to make sure no one is missed. Voice or text messages aren't sufficient.

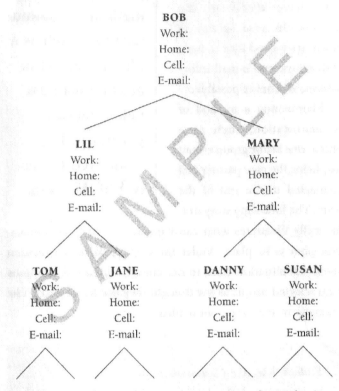

BOB
Work:
Home:
Cell:
E-mail:

LIL
Work:
Home:
Cell:
E-mail:

MARY
Work:
Home:
Cell:
E-mail:

TOM
Work:
Home:
Cell:
E-mail:

JANE
Work:
Home:
Cell:
E-mail:

DANNY
Work:
Home:
Cell:
E-mail:

SUSAN
Work:
Home:
Cell:
E-mail:

So, if Bob gets the first call, he calls Lil and Mary. But if, say, Lil isn't reachable, Bob calls Tom or Jane. It's important to keep this information current, so the name of the phone-tree coordinator (in this case, Bob) is on the sheet, too.

* This is a sample portion of a form you may wish to create or that will be found in our workbooks.

If you're using an e-mail group list, it's equally important to make sure each e-mail address is current. Ask for confirmation of receipt, since even the Internet isn't foolproof. And be sure to set up an alternate way of reaching those who don't have access to the Internet. In case service is down, it's a good idea to have both phone and e-mail information, whenever possible.

> Maintaining a method of communication, such as a phone tree list or group e-mail list, helps the care partner feel connected to the rest of the team.

Maintaining a method of communication, such as a phone tree list or group e-mail list, helps the care partner feel connected to the rest of the team. The following story dramatically illustrates what can happen when no communication plan is in place. Violet intended to keep information about her situation close to her chest, sharing only portions with selected people as she thought they needed to know. The dramatic results were unintended.

Violet's Selective Communication

Violet received the information that her cancer had returned with her characteristic determination and denial. She could tolerate only those people who would support her in looking toward a completely renewed healthy future, and so she shared only pieces of her medical situation with most people. She had created her own care-share team, made up of individuals who, for the most part, didn't know, or even know of, the others. Violet didn't trust that these friends or associates would be at her side if they met one another or knew the full story. She feared that if they met each other they'd form friendships and would abandon her. Her sense of safety kept her operating as the hub of a wheel with her team members scattered along the rim, separated from one another by the absence of any roster, meeting, or overlap.

This worked out all right while Violet was mostly able to live at home. It all fell apart, however, when she was hospitalized a few months before the end of her life. With no one holding Health Care Power of Attorney, doctors were unable to inform anyone about her wishes. The hospital confidentiality policies and the Health Insurance Portability and Accountability Act of 1996 (HIPAA) prevented friends from visiting her on the intensive care ward. Several of those who had actually been quite close to her didn't even know what was going on or where to find their friend, because no one else knew of her relationships. They were concerned and fearful on her behalf, yet had no way to get information. At the end, Violet was quite alone.

For this team there was no closure. Weeks went by until a distant relative came forward to sort through Violet's things. This person found names of her care team and pieced together the story. The group, however, never did coalesce.

HONOR YOUR COMMITMENTS

Remember, it's important that team members take their commitments seriously. Sticking with tasks and schedules creates a safety net for the care partner. Unfulfilled promises and unfinished tasks have a negative impact on the care partner's life and force another team member to pick up the pieces. As Alexander Pope said, "To err is human, to forgive, divine," but because this is probably a time when nerves are a bit frayed all around, it's wise not to ask for too much on the divine level from human compatriots. It's best to let others know as early as possible if a commitment can't be honored, for whatever reason.

> Sticking with tasks and schedules creates a safety net for the care partner.

Although commitment is important, so too is flexibility. However, if you're considering whether or not to participate, or whether or not to include a specific individual, it's important to speak to the issue of taking on only those tasks or times that are truly going to work, as best as you can foresee. Each person will have different amounts of time, skills, and areas of expertise. Some may volunteer on a daily basis, others once a week, still others every month or "on call." In some cases team members may provide professional backup to mediate, give counsel, or encourage. Other members may call, or pray, or send love. What's important to remember is that all contributions matter.

> What's important to remember is that all contributions matter.

Evaluate how much you, or others, can commit to a potential care team. You need to be clear, in your own mind and with others, how much and how often you can offer help. Schedules, cell phones, and computers can help the team keep in touch, but no tool will help if you simply don't follow through.

BUILD TRUST

We like respected psychologist Dr. Oscar G. Mink's definition of trust: "A person's confident expectation that another person's behavior will be consistently responsive and supportive to the mutual interests of both persons." Trust has also been defined as confidence in and reliance on good qualities, especially fairness, truth, honor, ability, or responsibility. However you define it, trust is important in a care-share environment. You can build trust by being consistent in doing what you've promised, maintaining confidentiality, and remembering to focus on your care partner's needs. Having a sense of humor, taking care of oneself spiritually and physically, and bringing difficulties regarding caregiving to the group will all deepen trust.

Trust: "A person's confident expectation that another person's behavior will be consistently responsive and supportive to the mutual interests of both persons."

For the care partner, trusting in the people who have come together to help him can be, surprisingly, a challenge. This kind of relationship may be new: Relying on others in ways you never even imagined can be hard. For example, if your care partner's world has been reduced because of mobility issues, people who are late can cause him great anxiety. He may question your loyalty and wonder if you even care. Having someone drop a task, even unintentionally, may raise doubts and fears. If someone questions his preferences or offers a different point of view, he may feel attacked. Learning to trust will take time.

Forming a "perfect" trust among care-share team members can be tricky— and humanly unlikely.

Forming a "perfect" trust among care-share team members can be tricky—and humanly unlikely. But discussing problems openly, acknowledging mistakes, keeping a sense of humor close at hand, and recognizing that we all do things differently are important ingredients for building trust among team members. Equally important is having a clear understanding of who is going to do what and when. Once trust is broken, it can be hard to reestablish, especially if it goes unmentioned. Trust should be held gently.

ENTER CAREFULLY INTO SOMEONE ELSE'S LIFE

It always seems like a sacred invitation and act of trust when a person allows you to come within the boundaries and borders of her life. Respectfully acknowledge what an act of courage is being made when your care partner opens her more personal, private life and needs, vulnerabilities and fears, hopes and dreams. You are a guest in her private world. Be careful, go slowly, and honor this special circumstance.

Acknowledge the sacred trust not only of the care partner, but also of her family. Every family has its own shape and dynamics. When you, as a nonfamily team member, enter

> You are a guest in her private world. Be careful, go slowly, and honor this special circumstance.

into this complicated realm, it's because you are needed. There is much you don't know about this family. And, while you're a valued team member, you're still not privy to years of history. It's important that you, as a team member, try not to judge or to fix families nor get into the middle of complex family interactions. The family will most likely welcome you—and the care partner's life will be enhanced—if you are respectful and supportive, but not invasive. Let trust build gradually. Ideally, you and the care partner will have been in the same safety net for years, experiencing the give and take of personal communication and establishing a respectful intimacy.

TAKE CARE OF YOURSELF

We cannot give what we do not have. A Native American saying reminds us, "You cannot give someone a drink from an empty cup." When you help someone, even though you might be glad to do so, the effort can be demanding, especially if there is no apparent improvement. Don't

> Life is to live—have a good time at it!

be surprised to be occasionally emotionally drained through the effort. It's also true that the effort of helping another is enriching and rewarding—so how can we find the balance? Below we've reprinted the advice of some retired residents of Providence

Mount St. Vincent, a wonderful continuing care facility in Seattle, Washington. There the residents are encouraged to look beyond themselves to the needs of others. This is their wisdom—how they charge their helping batteries—as it was submitted to their in-house newsletter:

- Understand that everything has a purpose: Be curious and discover it!
- Make time for a friend, even if you're tired.
- Find a way to stay productive: Someone has a need just for you to help with.
- A smile is ageless.
- Take time to really look in someone's eyes and just enjoy the quiet.
- Be grateful for the blessing of wonderful people in your life, even when they pass on.
- Have faith in God's plan.
- All the trivial experiences will pass by; what's important will stay with you.
- Be amazed at what you can do.
- Life is to live—have a good time of it!

(This list was published in Living, Summer 2004.)

Experiment and figure out how to recharge your own batteries: be it a walk in the woods, a raucous concert, or the smile of a baby. No matter if you are the caregiver or receiver, take time for nourishing yourself.

RESPECT BOUNDARIES AND ROLES

One common way you, as a caregiver, can get overwhelmed is by forgetting to take care of yourself. If the care partner's needs become so paramount that your own personal needs are ignored, problems will surely follow. Boundaries (or limits) and roles are tricky and subtle. Boundaries are too loose when care team members proceed beyond or behave outside specified and agreed upon roles and the behavior appropriate to that role. For example, if a paid younger caregiver begins acting like a daughter, with corresponding expectations for maternal solicitude from the older woman she cares for, this young woman would be violating a boundary. Or the converse would be true if the older woman gives advice, money, or gifts to the younger caregiver, as she would to her own daughters.

Entering into a care-share team can be somewhat like going into a foreign country. You will need to try to understand and respect the expectations, sensitivities, customs, and needs of the care partner and his family system. Sometimes the care partner or someone who knows him well can help. Sometimes the team may need the assistance of a translator or counselor. But unless these rules are communicated, no one will be able to follow them. Awareness, curiosity, and respect will help the whole team understand the boundaries of this new land.

Sometimes boundaries and roles, rather than being forgotten, are too firmly and rigidly held. An example of this might be when a friend joins a care-share team and performs her responsibilities in an overly crisp, businesslike, even cold fashion, focusing only on the task at hand without showing compassion to the care partner. Caring for feelings and each other's hearts is imperative.

How do you know when you're approaching a boundary line? What's just on this side? What's on the other side? How do you stop? If only personal boundary lines were as easy to discern as property boundary lines: You could get a survey and know for certain. But personal boundary lines relate to subtle— sometimes intangible—issues

> Be quick to communicate, to apologize, and to correct your course of action.

such as personal space, privacy, body functions, religious beliefs, family relationships, and deeply held hopes and fears. We believe you should go slowly. Be quick to communicate, to apologize, and to correct your course of action. This is new territory, where you all work together to discover what works and feels right and what doesn't. Make the needed changes along the way. Your personal growth and increased connections will be your reward.

A friend shared this story about struggling with boundaries. Her compassion for her friend had brought her dangerously close to a personal edge of fatigue, discord with her husband, and emotional distress.

Only Friends

"Will you be my friend?" has been a defining question of mine since I was little, maybe three or four years old. Though I've never had dozens and dozens of friends, I've predictably had a handful, and treasured each for her or his gifts and place in my life. I can't remember ever having a "best" friend, even in grade school, when such alliances were common, and commonly endangered. I've always had a few very good friends, though. Many times these friends were in turn someone else's best friend.

So, it was with some sense of alarm that I heard my care partner refer to me as her best friend, her only friend. What could this mean? What about my husband, the closest friend I'd ever had, who, though supportive of my role in my friend's life, also wanted more of my time? It raised a level of anxiety that I neither welcomed nor understood. I struggled with a sense of confusion and dismay.

The idea of her being a best or only friend to me, I discovered, was accompanied by feeling overwhelmed and engulfed by the personality, needs, and complexities of my care partner. Through many conversations with her and some counseling, I came to see that what she intended was a testimony to our growing fondness for each other. She "labeled" our relationship this way so that she could freely ask for help from me. But I felt it was a scary weight. I learned that throughout her life she had customarily had one "best" friend, clearly a foreign concept to me. Moreover, it was my problem, and one of boundaries.

After several weeks of prayer, journaling, and talking with a counselor, I became clear with myself, and then with her. While I could not be comfortable at all with the thought of being an "only friend," I could be delighted to be her best friend, as long as she understood that I could not reciprocate. Meaning no disrespect to her, I simply wasn't about to relinquish myself to having only one friend, or even one best friend.

Through all of this, I learned that while I can be a very, very good friend, I cannot be an even adequate only friend: It's simply not something I can do. Thank heavens she could understand and accept what I was saying and what I could offer.

PLAY AND REJUVENATE

What do an ice cream social, a silly white elephant gift exchange, May Day flowers, and brown bag picnics have in common? They are ways in which teams can have some fun while celebrating their partnership. Monthly potluck dinners fall into the same category and allow teams to socialize and take care of business. Other teams we've known celebrate birthdays, go bowling, or create collages. Get creative with your team and decide what would serve your needs.

> Playing and rejuvenating will help balance the team's perspective, even in the midst of inevitable frustrations and tensions.

Mental health is improved if there is a focus on something or someone else and if there is laughter in life. Being part of a safety net by participating in a care-share team definitely provides the opportunity to focus on others. And playing and rejuvenating will help balance the team's perspective, even in the midst of inevitable frustrations and tensions.

KEEP RITUALS AND TRADITIONS

Rituals, traditions, and ceremonies also help maintain a positive balance in the emotions of a team. You can create rituals around welcoming someone new into a team, opening or closing meetings, saying good-bye to a team member, or periodically celebrating the group's ongoing existence.

Gathering visual or mental images, writing group thank-you notes, burning papers that represent resentments or good memories—these efforts channel emotions in positive directions. Art can open the heart: Capturing memories with a note, photo, picture, collage, or piece of artwork is one way to start. Water represents renewal and cleansing. Fire is purifying and signals letting go to a higher power or the universe. Sharing food is a common gesture of welcome and trust.

Rituals can also function as a way—even a habit—of acknowledging the contributions of team members: Set aside time at each meeting to say something positive about the other team members. Give each person the "floor" for a few moments during every meeting to report on how things are going. Post a photo board of names and faces, and list ways each person has pitched in. The idea here is to clearly identify what each person has contributed and celebrate it.

> Clearly identify what each person has contributed and celebrate it.

Some people use rituals and ceremonies to say good-bye to their homes—or their independence. In the following story, a counselor tells us how Rita used a bittersweet ceremony as she left her much-loved home and moved to an assisted living facility.

Rita's Good-Bye to Her Home

Into the first room we went, Rita in her electric wheelchair and me following her. Rita slowly scanned the room with her camcorder. Tears rolled down her cheeks as she began to speak. She described first seeing the house, then deciding that it would work given her growing disability, and finally making it into a home—her home.

Now it was time to say good-bye. Moving from room to room, she repeated the following ritual: She read a short thank-you to each room for its service to her over the years; then she lit the note with a candle, burned it to ash, and added the ash to the potted plant she would take to the assisted living facility that would be her next home. She lingered in her craft room, where she had spent many hours in the creative process, making gifts for others. It had been an important and fulfilling form of self-expression. We circled back to the living room where we had enjoyed many cups of tea and meaningful conversations.

She thanked me for accompanying her on yet another leg of her journey. She seemed at peace and ready to say her final good-bye to this home she had loved.

GET READY

Communicate:	Set up a system and try it out. Occasionally ask team members how it's working. Tweak as needed.
Acknowledge:	Make it a practice to thank each other for the work accomplished on behalf of the care partner.
Remember:	Take time to laugh and play.
Be brave:	Look in the mirror and say out loud three statements that you feel strongly about but find it hard to say to the person who needs to hear them, such as, "I'm angry about missing my own family dinner when Susie doesn't show up on time," or "I'm scared to be with Mitch when his parents aren't around." Sometimes just saying these things aloud takes away their power. Speak your message with feeling.
Be productive:	Keep meetings brief. Agree upon a schedule. Stick to ground rules. Try out ideas.
Pay attention:	Do you feel good about your involvement? Take care of yourself, too.

CHAPTER 6
Know What to Expect

Whether you have formed a care-share team for yourself or for someone else—or even if you're just contemplating whether to join a team—you can realistically assume that there will be surprises ahead. When you're part of someone's personal safety net, try to plan as best you can, but prepare for the unexpected. You may find yourself protecting the care partner's privacy, feeling intense emotions, fighting stress and burnout, or simply wanting more time for yourself.

> Plan as best you can, but prepare for the unexpected.

LOSS OF PRIVACY

It's always hard to give up or share privacy. As a potential caregiver, you can be very sensitive and respectful of the care partner's personal space. Keep in mind that the care partner's privacy needs may ebb and flow based on treatments, fluctuating feelings of vulnerability, and other factors.

Catherine Protects Benjamin's Privacy

Catherine knew she needed help caring for her husband of sixty-two years. She and her husband enjoyed strong bonds with several close friends, including their next-door neighbor, Alice. Both friends and neighbors were eager to help this wonderful couple as soon as they heard of the need, but Catherine was worried that their help might compromise Benjamin's needs for privacy. Benjamin was a retired physician and Catherine a wonderful musician. They were cultured, proper, and well mannered in the style of the country from which they had immigrated.

Benjamin had suffered a major stroke. Although he had completed nine months of rehabilitation, he had not recovered his ability to speak or use one arm and one leg. He needed help with many personal tasks.

As days passed and Catherine came to acknowledge how tired she'd become, she finally agreed to let their neighbor, Alice, help. Alice was a gifted and sensitive physical therapist and knew to treat Benjamin with the utmost respect, to always maintain his personal modesty in even the smallest of ways, and to express what an honor it was to give back to a man who had given so much to so many people. Catherine could tell that Benjamin liked Alice and was able to accept her careful entry into his personal and private space. With time Catherine and

Alice brought, one by one, more friends to join in a care-share team. Catherine thanked Alice for her sensitivity and "way" with Benjamin. Alice talked with each new team member about what she had learned in helping Benjamin be comfortable receiving help. Most importantly, Benjamin's life was enhanced by increased, sensitive interactions.

It's often difficult to figure out how to speak sensitively and act respectfully once privacy needs are known. At issue may be the care partner's physical needs (such as speaking on the phone without being overheard, or bathing) or emotional needs (knowing the details of her life won't be shared with anyone else). Even if the care partner is unable to talk about such issues, team members can help one another.

> Often, in times of crisis or great stress, people act out of fear.

DIFFICULT FEELINGS FOR EVERYONE

One of the more challenging and, at times, rewarding aspects of sharing care involves dealing with the various and sometimes new feelings you may experience. Often, in times of crisis or great stress, people act out of fear. A friend tells this story about Brigitte, suggesting that her fears guided her actions.

Brigitte's Story

My friend Brigitte didn't tell me she was being admitted into the hospital. Though she had once talked about creating a list of who was helping her, this never happened, and I don't think many of her friends had actually met each other. After days of worry, I finally found out that she was in the hospital, so I went to see her. I told her that I had felt worried and alone when I didn't know where she was. Brigitte, in turn, admitted her fear that if those involved in assisting her knew one another, they'd bond together and leave her. I replied that it was more likely that we'd support one another in helping her. But she was unconvinced.

You may dismiss Brigitte's extreme fear and think, "I wouldn't have that fear." However, being a sensitive member of a care-share team requires tuning in to the unique person whose life has now changed and who is trying to find stability in this foreign and often frightening territory of change or illness. If you are caring for a relative or close friend, you may feel you know that person well and know what to expect. But this is not always true. Adopting a curious, open, and accepting attitude toward how a friend or loved one will respond in this new territory can be very valuable.

The following is a partial list of some of the commonly reported feelings that we two authors in our various professional and personal experiences have witnessed or personally felt. When reading this list try to imagine what it would be like to have this feeling. Do not judge it, but rather experience it. This will help you prepare for a time when this feeling may arise in you or another team member. If it is you who is the care partner, then take comfort in knowing that others have felt exactly how you feel.

> Adopting a curious, open, and accepting attitude toward how a friend or loved one will respond in this new territory can be very valuable.

INTENSE EMOTIONS

- **Numbness/Denial**: "I can't believe this happened to me"; not wanting this to be real; seeing a small improvement as major hope; thinking "I'll get well."
- **Fear**: "I can't do this," or "I don't know what to expect."
- **Suspense**: "When will I get well?" or "When will I die?" or "When will I hear the things I've always wanted to hear?"
- **Anger**: at the illness, at siblings for not helping more, at watching money dwindle, at feeling helpless, at the disruption in life, at the unfairness.

- **Guilt**: for feeling anger, for not doing more, for not taking better care of myself, for burdening others, for being sick, for needing help, for not being able to bear or alleviate the pain, indignity, or humiliation.

- **Compassion**: for both myself and others, as we cope with needs, pain, impatience, or grief.

- **Grief and sadness**: for dreams that may never come true, for relationships that will never be the same, for missed opportunities, for a future that now seems shorter.

- **Regret**: for what wasn't said, for time not taken, for dreams not realized.

- **Shame**: for wishing to die, for not always saying thanks, for not always giving wonderful loving care, for getting sick in the first place.

- **Embarrassment**: for my appearance or behavior, for not having it all together.

- **Joy**: for all that my life has meant or brought to others, for small tokens of love or affection, for seeing an end to the suffering and exhaustion.

- **Powerlessness**: nothing will make a difference, not being able to bring comfort, not being able to "solve this problem," not being able to do and give in the old ways.

- **Burnout**: for too many demands, too few breaks, too little coming into one's life, the medical demands.

- **Protectiveness**: of our loved one, of ourselves, of our ideas, of how things ought to be.

- **Laughter**: Sometimes the tremendous stress and tension can be relieved through humor. It's wonderful! Don't be embarrassed or shy about it or the intensity with which you laugh. You need it, too!

- **Confusion**: in the face of any or all of the above, often intensified by fatigue and feeling overwhelmed.

This may be a time to take a break from reading this book. Many people find the "emotional rehearsal" of trying on these various feelings very tiring. It is hard work, but may leave you better prepared for the emotional demands of caregiving or care receiving. It is helpful if you can talk with others along the way. It's comforting to know you are in the company of others who care. In the following story, a sensitive man reflects back on the conflicted emotions he experienced as a young man who helped care for his mother.

A Family Reacts to Nellie's Stroke

It was 1967. I distinctly remember sitting in a booth at the small country cafe *where our family was well known. It had been over two years since Mom's massive stroke, and there had been little recovery. One aftermath of her stroke was that she could not eat without spilling food all over herself. The stroke also left her with the strange quality of starting a sentence but then skipping from topic to topic without stopping. Whoever she was talking with was then held captive for long periods of time. My sister was then eighteen, I was twenty, and Dad was forty-three. As much as we all loved Mom, we were also wrestling with our feelings. We felt protective of Mom, but we also felt embarrassed: She had taught us impeccable table manners that she herself could no longer follow. We struggled with powerlessness to make it all better despite all our efforts, prayers, and conversations with health-care professionals.*

We felt anger that things were so different compared to before Mom's stroke. Tenderness, love, and compassion were there as well as we sat with this innocent and vulnerable person, our mom, who now relied on us for her care and well-being.

Delving into the many ways you can come to grips with feelings as a care partner or as a caregiver is beyond the scope and intention of this book. Yet you must recognize and manage feelings and reactions. Many people find help through friends, family, clergy, or support groups, and others choose to consult with a counselor specially trained in this area. Many books in the Bibliography offer excellent guidance. We encourage you to talk, read, consult, pray, or process in as many ways that make sense to you.

Far too many husbands, wives, adult children, partners, and occasionally friends, out of love and responsibility, provide more care than they can physically and emotionally sustain. This often happens because they have not created a safety net and are used to being very self-reliant and independent. Or it happens because they think of their loved one as the only person needing help. But this can be heartbreaking to watch. We've seen well-meaning loved ones jeopardize their own health, sometimes even their own lives, by putting another's needs so exclusively ahead of their own. This usually happens slowly, until one day, a caregiver burns out, experiences a health crisis, or uncharacteristically loses his temper and lashes out at the care partner. Remember how Catherine, in this chapter's first story, recognized her need for help in time? Beth, in the story below, takes longer.

> Talk, read, consult, pray, or process in as many ways that make sense to you.

Beth's Story

Beth was fifty-nine. She lovingly cared for her seventy-eight-year-old husband, Harry, whose Alzheimer's disease had progressed to the point where he could no longer remember his age. He became confused and agitated in the late afternoon, insisting on going for a walk and feeling upset when he couldn't remember where he was. His twenty-three-year-old daughter regularly stopped by so Beth could run errands and shop. Eventually Harry began waking in the night, going outside, and heading off. Beth, exhausted and frail, had lost weight, neglected her health, and feared she might be developing even higher blood pressure. She was too busy to go see her own physician. During one especially frightening night, Harry walked off and could not be found until early morning when the police brought him home. There they found Beth on the floor. She had suffered a stroke.

Beth's dramatic story is all too common. It underscores the critical need for care teams to support *all* members so that no one single person carries too heavy a load. Also, care sharing allows the primary loved ones—whether spouse, son or daughter, partner, or friend—to rest, take good care of themselves, and maintain connection with the rest of their lives. They then have much more to give during the time they are with their loved one.

BURNOUT

Recognizing and setting personal boundaries is one helpful way to avoid getting overwhelmed or experiencing burnout, which is feeling empty and having nothing left to give. To help your care partner maintain the best quality of life possible, it's important to sustain the good function of yourself and your team. Primary or solitary caregivers are notoriously overworked, under-recognized, under-supported, isolated, and likely to suffer from burnout. But team members, too, can become overtaxed. While good communication, well-thought-out care plans, and many outside resources can help stave off burnout, only you can prevent it. It is important to learn to recognize the signs of burnout—both in yourself and in the other team members—and take a break, when needed.

> Care-sharing allows the primary loved ones—whether spouse, son or daughter, partner, or friend—to rest, take good care of themselves, and maintain connection with the rest of their lives.

Burnout refers to feeling as though there is "nothing left to give"—emotionally, physically, mentally, spiritually, or all of the above. The well is empty. Stress contributes to burnout. So do environmental factors, such as working conditions, home life, or health. Burnout generally occurs over time, although the related symptoms may seem to occur overnight.

People experience burnout in varying degrees of intensity and duration: Some feel a lack of energy. Some wish to escape entirely. Some constantly struggle with the effects of burnout. As a caregiver's struggle continues, burnout threatens physical, mental, and emotional health. You can recognize the signs of burnout and take corrective action before it is too late. We have compiled the list below to help you recognize these signs and prevent you from being drawn into this state, which jeopardizes your health and your ability to offer care.

> Primary or solitary caregivers are notoriously overworked, under-recognized, under-supported, isolated, and likely to suffer from burnout.

SYMPTOMS OF BURNOUT

- I no longer participate in the activities I used to enjoy.
- I feel blue, irritable, hopeless, and helpless more often than not.
- I find myself getting upset more quickly than normal.
- I am getting sick more often than normal.

- I feel like I can't take it one more day.

- I feel overwhelmed and fantasize about escape.

- I want to hurt the person I am caring for.

- I want to hurt myself.

- I have a low frustration tolerance.

- I feel futile, and at a loss for meaning and purpose.

- I feel emotionally exhausted and spiritually bankrupt.

- I feel depressed.

- I am being more moody than usual.

- I have less patience.

- I am emotionally withdrawing and having fewer contacts with friends.

- I am experiencing more difficulty sleeping.

- I worry more.

- I am expressing a more negative attitude than usual.

- I feel more apathetic.

- I feel more cynical.

- I feel overwhelmed.

- I want to distance myself from the team.

If you're feeling burnt out, you may find it helpful to consult with a professional counselor who specializes in the unique stresses and strains that go with caregiving. Or you could use the following list to help you stop or slow your growing burnout:

- Are your expectations of what you can do realistic? Do you need to shift them?

- Do you need to get better at saying no and at setting limits to protect yourself, your time, your energy?

- Do you need to know more about the illness, disease, surgery, and situation?

- Can you ask for help? Remember *help appeal* and practice asking for help. In workshops we often practice asking for help because it's so foreign and so hard for many of us.

- Would you benefit from developing and using both your team and your personal safety net?

- Are you taking breaks? The sooner the better. Many caregivers complain that it's a hassle to arrange substitute care. We suggest you make taking breaks part of your routine; you can build your "days off" right into the schedule, and other members can learn to cover for you.

- Is it time to learn a stress management technique? Find a great book, audiotape, or workshop. Pick one, learn it, use it, and it will help keep you healthy and de-stressed in all aspects of your life.

- Call a counselor or consultant who is an expert on what you're experiencing.

Jody, in the next story, turns to a professional care manager when she's at her wit's end. Her story is told from the care manager's perspective. It holds out hope for those of you who are exhausted.

Jody: Care Plan for the Caregiver

Jody had wanted to consult with me about her forty-six-year-old husband whose battle with cancer was in its second year. He had become increasingly withdrawn and emotionally closed off. She and their late-adolescent children were concerned and missed his personality and emotional presence. They'd heard that I could be helpful to men dealing with serious illness. While, as a counselor and coach, I believed I could help him recover some emotional solid footing, my first concern was Jody.

She looked and sounded exhausted. While she was telling me about her husband, his illness, his treatments, and how hard all of this had been for him, I was able to extract some information about her. After assuring her that I would meet with her husband, I turned my attention to her. She had many of the symptoms of burnout, and she confessed to not having seen her own doctor and dentist for her annual check-ups and to numerous other examples of self-neglect.

Our time had run out and I agreed to meet with her husband on one condition: that together we develop two related plans. One plan would be for her, to help her regain her health and reduce her load. A second plan would be for a care-share team, which would be valuable both to her husband and to the rest of the family. She trusted me, we met, and we created both plans. With many modifications over the next several months, our plans supported the family to the end of their difficult journey.

NEEDING TIME FOR YOURSELF

Part of Jody's care plan for herself was establishing her own boundaries or limits. Besides sharing the concerns and care for her husband with a team, she also learned to take time for herself.

Loraine's Tale

Loraine had always been the beautiful belle around whom all the others flocked. She was always ready for a party or an adventure. Tim fell madly in love with her, paying no attention at all when she told him of her progressive disease that would probably claim her life early. What could that matter to him when he loved her so much?

Years went by, and the disease did make inroads. Loraine's ability to move about dwindled alarmingly. Pain became her constant companion. She was forced to follow a complicated medication schedule. Tim was Loraine's main caregiver, yet he was also holding down a job—and feeling more and more overwhelmed. Even when they hired caregivers for daytime help, Tim's evenings were always slated to care for Loraine.

Tim didn't mind at first. He gladly did what was needed. As time went on, however, and the bubbly and competent woman he'd married became bedridden and pain filled, Tim's own inner resources were stretched thin. He didn't see how he could get any relief and became resentful. Yet being angry seemed wrong to him somehow, when Loraine was so ill. Concerned friends offered to help, but Tim declined.

One night, Tim just didn't come home. On another night he "went for a drive" and drove to the next state, not returning until the wee hours. On a third night, he took Loraine with him, but left her medicines behind. Tim was acting out his frustrations and feelings in a way that really endangered Loraine.

For her part, Loraine covered for Tim. She told caregivers who arrived in the morning that she'd just overslept and that was why she'd not been to the bathroom. Doctors questioned whether Loraine was taking the proper dosages of prescribed medications after their effectiveness decreased. Finally, someone reached the conclusion that Tim needed help, too.

Unfortunately, by the time Tim received this offer of

assistance, his relationship with Loraine was beyond repair. The trust had been broken irrevocably. It would have been so much better if Tim had invited others to help him care for his wife sooner. Though neighbors and friends had offered, he hadn't acknowledged his own inadequacies and therefore was unable to accept help. In trying to go it alone, he put Loraine in danger, as well.

When the group stepped in to help, Lorraine stopped denying her need. Tim, ashamed and frustrated, left the house. Although their confusing scenario ended in divorce, in the end Lorraine received better care and lived for many more years.

Like Tim, many people only learn the hard way to know and respect individual limits. Then it can be too late. Asking for and accepting help before there's a crisis is a huge favor for all involved. In the next story Gary seeks help just in time.

Gary's Final Straw

Phyllis had been disabled for many years by a massive stroke and then congestive heart failure. Gary, her seventy-year-old husband, was exhausted and burnt out by the combination of caregiving and operating his farm. For several years his doctor had been insisting that Gary take some time off, but he just didn't see how he could. A source of strength for Gary was a close friend, Phil, who was also caring for his own wife. While they loved their wives, the strain of solo caregiving had gotten to be too much. Gary and Phil both imagined a time when their loved ones would pass on and they could retire with time and energy for some pleasurable activities with other family and friends. Then Gary's friend unexpectedly died of a heart attack. Gary was grief stricken and brought to his knees by both the loss of his friend and the shattering of his dream and hope for shared time later.

Only when Gary became seriously depressed did he ask for help from others, who came together as a care-share team. A niece, who was director of nursing at a nearby nursing home, arranged temporary care for Phyllis. Gary took a long overdue vacation to Florida to walk the beaches, nap in the sun, and visit with relatives there. For the first time in years, he relaxed, free of pressures and responsibilities. Two weeks later Gary returned, rested, healed, and ready to resume his responsibilities for the remaining seven months of his wife's life. For these months, however, both he and his wife were supported by his niece, family, and friends.

As a caregiver, you may be so busy performing daily tasks that you forget to check in with yourself and assess your emotional, physical, and spiritual well-being. As hard as it may sound, setting aside some time each day to sit in a quiet place and turn attention inward can help charge your care-giving batteries.

> As hard as it may sound, setting aside some time each day to sit in a quiet place and turn attention inward can help charge your care-giving batteries.

Some people meditate during this time. Others take a walk or retreat to a special place in the home or a favorite cafe or park bench where they feel at peace. Exercise is another powerful antidote. Whether you take half an hour or half a day off from caregiving responsibilities, the time should help clear both your mind and your spirit.

Spend a few moments assessing your situation and honestly determining if it is time to seek more support. Be realistic: It takes a whole community to support a care partner—that is what the care-share team is created to do. Don't worry yet about how or where help will come from. What's important now is taking even

> It's best to address the problems before they develop into a crisis.

small signs of emotional distress seriously. It's best to address the problems before they develop into a crisis.

Once you've arranged for extra help in caregiving, you will find that you have time to focus on other interests. It is critical to have activities in your life that renew you and leave you with added vigor and energy. These vary from person to person, of course, but it's important for you to discover what renews you and pursue it. It is important for you as well as your care partner.

With adequate care support, you'll also have time for other important relationships in your life. All relationships require attention, and because caregiving can be incredibly time consuming, often the entire family suffers the loss of the primary caregiver's

> Reaffirming other relationships can have wonderful, revitalizing results—and will actually enhance caregiving abilities.

focus and energy. Friendships will have lapsed as well. Reaffirming other relationships can have wonderful, revitalizing results—and will actually enhance caregiving abilities. By involving a care-share team, the members can help one another remember their individual needs for boundaries, balance, and self-care.

LIFE AS A MEDICAL PROBLEM

With a serious or life-threatening illness, your life may seem to be primarily a medical problem. How will this affect my ability to visit my children or grandchildren? Can I go to work? Can I get to the grocery store? Can I watch TV? Will my retirement be what we had hoped and saved to make it? This perspective is often colored when you're undergoing a medical test. What will the test show? What happens if it is positive? When waiting for medical test results, which can take days and days, you may simply put your life on hold; you're unable to focus on anything else.

You may worry that, from the outside, this looks terribly self-absorbed and even selfish. But you also know, inside, you are facing fears and uncertainties, and your mind and attention are being taken over by the illness. Both push what used to be "normal" away and often increase your sense of isolation from close family and friends.

Tina's World Got Smaller and "Medicalized"

Tina's world began to shrink as her disease process continued. More and more of her time and energy became focused on doctor's appointments, visits from home-health nurses, and the difficulty of performing simple tasks. Fewer and fewer things outside of this immediate realm interested her. Most of the people Tina interacted with wanted to know about her health. Her energy level seldom could be sustained beyond responding to their queries. "How are you feeling?" replaced "What do you think about that guy who was elected to our school board?"

Tina's close friends and family would probably not admit it, but their image of Tina was shifting from mother, sister, and friend to "the sick one." The shift eliminated any common ground needed for relationships to flourish. People drifted away, and Tina felt more isolated.

Then Tina broke her ankle. Because of all the stairs in her home, she needed to recover in a rehabilitation facility. This intensified not only the focus on health and healing but also Tina's "medicalization." She became a "good" patient: She presented more symptoms, more problems. She was "interesting" to the doctors and nurses, who regularly checked on their "poor" patient. The attention increased with more need, and to a certain extent was appropriate and good.

Fewer and fewer people came to visit Tina. And as her mobility declined, her weight increased. Eventually her ankle healed and she returned home, but moving about became even more difficult. She needed more help with her care than ever, and moving to a nursing facility seemed to be the next logical step.

During her stay in the nursing facility, Tina's symptoms multiplied and she saw fewer and fewer visitors. Outside circumstances required Tina to move yet again, and her situation was beginning to seem hopeless. That's when a skilled therapist entered her life. With newfound vision, will, and hope, and the guidance of her therapist, Tina chose to move into a hybrid assisted living/boarding house. Family and caregivers couldn't imagine what would become of her.

What happened next, however, was a testimony to Tina's inner strength. In a setting with more real-life activities and a broader spectrum of people about her, Tina's self-image improved. She slowly shifted her focus away from her symptoms and toward the needs of the other residents— especially to newcomers. While she did not return to full health, she did begin to make new friends and become more interested in others, and, in turn, more interesting. Her "medicalization" appeared to be in remission. Perhaps it would not return.

An illness means a new set of characters will enter your life. In one respect, you may view these doctors, nurses, and insurance representatives as unwelcome intruders. You may just wish they would all go away. In another respect, however, these new folks are the people who will help you heal and enter this new phase of life. Each of them is a gift. They provide understanding and knowledge, deliver needed treatments, and may notice small but significant changes that will help you cope. And while their roles are important, they may not understand or be able to deal with all the emotional issues involved. It's wise to try to prepare for this.

> These new folks are the people who will help you heal and enter this new phase of life.

They react with their own hopes, fears, preferences, and opinions, which may or may not be compatible with yours.

LACK OF STABILITY

You may question how to respond to these new people who have now taken such important roles in your life. Your first reaction may be to dismiss them. Another reaction is to comply unquestioningly to their directions, but this can make things even worse. Those patients who often fare the best are those who see themselves as in charge of their own health and who view their physicians as critical team members. Being feisty, making personal decisions with a lot of input, and not necessarily pleasing everyone seem to be life giving and health promoting. These characteristics help you take control and thereby decrease your anxiety. Even small steps matter. It is often through first experiencing and then dealing with emotional reactions that you develop your emotional solid footing.

> Being feisty, making personal decisions with a lot of input, and not necessarily pleasing everyone seem to be life-giving and health promoting.

It is okay to question, get angry, and fight for life. With questioning comes understanding, with fight comes hope. It is important to question repeatedly, especially if frightened, anxious, or in pain. Repetition reinforces your understanding and helps you achieve the solid ground necessary for further discussions and treatments. Smart patients make conscious and repeated efforts to develop and use all inner and outer resources to find and re-find stability in this new world.

Wendall's Search for Emotional Stability

First the *symptoms, then the many doctors' visits and tests. It was all exhausting and frightening for Wendall. Having been through a lot of unexpected and unwelcome changes in his fifty-seven years, he believed himself to be quite resilient. Yet the diagnosis of an incurable cancer was way beyond his worst fear. Using all his knowledge, and that of many wise friends, he was able to minimize some fears, manage others, and continue many of his normal activities during the first few months. Some of his tactics to gain emotional stability included talking with his family and close friends, learning about his illness, and arranging for good medical care. He learned about alternative complementary health care, spent time in prayer, found solace and inspiration from others who had faced what he was now facing, and sought wisdom from caring counselors and consultants. Even with the intentional use of these strategies, and many more, Wendall still at times felt out of control, as if he was standing on shifting sand. Wendall realized that finding and re-finding stability amid these uncertainties would continuously challenge him. He often reminded himself that he was building a "road* map" for what was ahead. He had met and survived many challenges in his life thus far and trusted he would face and meet this one, too.

JUDGMENTS ABOUT ILLNESS

Serious or life-threatening illness can easily become public knowledge. Who can ignore in our neighbors or friends the visible signs of illness? Bandages, hair loss, crutches, and wheelchairs are clues to everyone that something is amiss. We are naturally curious to know what has happened. Even if the illness is not obvious, it often is known to our relatives and friends and subsequently many others in our lives. Who knows and doesn't know is often beyond our control.

Each person who finds out about someone's illness deals with it uniquely. Once a family member, friend, or colleague hears of an illness, questions arise: How did this happen? What does it mean for my friend? What does it mean for me? Why did this happen? There are a host of implications the illness might have on a relationship.

What happens to the information once it's shared is interesting, too. People's reactions depend as much on the meaning or beliefs they hold about the nature and cause of illness as it depends on what they're actually told, when they're told, or by whom.

> Mutual respect and appreciation of differing perspectives is often called for in a care-share team setting.

In his book *Grace and Grit*, Ken Wilber describes attitudes held by many major religions toward illness. Regardless of beliefs, perceptions of the cause of the problem can vary greatly even among friends and relatives. Understanding others' beliefs may help in tailoring responses to the problem and possible solutions. Mutual respect and appreciation of differing perspectives is often called for in a care-share team setting.

LOSS OF PERSPECTIVE

Finding, losing, and regaining perspective is an ongoing challenge whether you're giving or receiving care. And one of the deepest sources of pain for caregivers is guilt: "I promised him that I would never put him in a nursing home." "I promised him I'd protect his privacy by hiding his disability." "If I don't come by for at least two meals I can't be sure they'll feed him." "If I don't move in, he'll be sad, and then I'll feel guilty." "If I don't bail her out financially, her business will fail." Even when you really love the person you're caring for, the well

> You, too, may need a care plan to keep healthy and strong for the journey.

from which you are attempting to draw can be filled with frustration, guilt, and occasionally anger at a situation that may seem entirely unmanageable. Guilt and anger may cause you to completely lose your perspective. Sometimes the best way to really love your care partner is to create some distance in order to refill that well and rebuild resources. At times, it's not just the person with the "problem" who needs a care plan to guide him or her through what's ahead; you, too, may need a care plan to keep healthy and strong for the journey.

June Finds Her Wings

His diagnosis of cancer was totally unexpected. He was the pillar of health. They were both in their fifties and not at all prepared for the many challenges that would follow. One of the biggest worries was financial: While June was a working professional and had her own private business at which she was very good, the creative and expansive side of her did not find expression through her work. June countered the feeling of being both physically and financially trapped by developing a plan. By coincidence and good fortune, she and her husband had purchased a condo in the mountains the previous year, and June's creativity and expansiveness found wonderful expression through the remodel she designed and oversaw. June found renewed energy and stamina for dealing with her husband's situation through this creative outlet.

Following discussions with her husband and thoughtful conversations with friends and consultants, June decided to purchase a second condo, a fixer-upper to remodel and resell— with the hopes of making a handsome profit. As these things sometimes go, June's decision to take this risk, to "spread her wings" so to speak, was met with the perfect condo at a very good price. While June and her husband continued to face changes and challenges, June, in a very deep and important way, no longer felt trapped. She looked forward to taking on more projects where she could be creative and in charge. She, her husband, and a group of friends have created a strong team; the crisis, unexpectedly, helped her find her way back to hope and strength.

GET READY

Ask yourself: Is caregiving taking up a part of my life—or all of it? If it becomes the defining part, you're probably doing too much. Say so, and ask for some help.

Reflect: Try on various feelings. Which ones are you experiencing? You must first accept what you feel before you can address it. Acceptance leads to perspective.

Speak up: If you are experiencing any of the symptoms of burnout, say so. Get help as soon as possible.

Think: If you're receiving care, think about whether or not you are asking for what you need and receiving it in a way that feels helpful. If not, try to restate what you need at the next care-share meeting in a way that invites the help you want.

CHAPTER 7
Watch for Stumbling Blocks

Most of the problems encountered in care-share teams can be resolved. We believe it is helpful to learn about potential problems from the stories of other people's real-life dilemmas and how they solved them. As you expand your personal safety net, surround yourself with people who've had a broad range of experiences, ask them about their challenges, and learn from them. You will be better prepared to avoid or effectively deal with care-share problems if you can anticipate them. This chapter is our attempt to identify some stumbling blocks that we've most frequently encountered.

> As you expand your personal safety net, surround yourself with people who've had a broad range of experiences, ask them about their challenges, and learn from them.

EMOTIONAL TRAPS

You can expect that feelings of dependency will evoke strong emotions. People typically love to be needed, yet hate to be in need. "Needy" has such negative connotations that are hidden behind a pretense of having it all under control. We act as though having life under control means doing it all ourselves, or paying for help, but rarely asking for assistance. In the book *Still Here*, Ram Dass has observed that "being dependent, needing help, makes us feel diminished, because we value self-sufficiency and independence so highly. We value taking care of others, but shun the notion of being taken care of ourselves." You *can*, however, balance your independence with an ability to ask for help.

In addition, many of the emotions mentioned in earlier chapters are related to other "hot buttons," that, like dependency, are easily pushed: for example, guilt, fear, anger. Naming these takes away a lot of their power. Asking fellow team members for support in identifying when old patterns show up and in finding new ways to respond can help you avoid automatic responses.

Another trap is that of jealousy. You may feel your relationship with the care partner is threatened just by others forming a care team. This can be self-fulfilling.

Elizabeth and Her Daughter

Elizabeth needed help in taking care of her young daughter. A single mom with some serious health problems, Elizabeth was fiercely independent, though overwhelmed by parenting and considering putting her daughter up for adoption. Eventually, a school principal won Elizabeth's trust and supported her in seeking temporary foster care for the little girl. Another school family stepped up and received training and certification to become her foster parents. It should have been a big red flag that, at this point, Elizabeth dragged her heels in actually placing her daughter in the official foster care system, as she had agreed upon. This was the first time Elizabeth would act counter to agreements, and it was a passive-aggressive response to her unacknowledged fears and jealousy. Instead of speaking of these and enlisting even more support from a team, Elizabeth pushed for the girl to immediately live with the foster family "until the process was complete." The truth was that Elizabeth feared that her daughter would thrive in the new family system and even love her less as she came to love the new family more. The family, with reservations about this sequence, nevertheless agreed to take in the girl, even though she wasn't officially registered in the foster-care system.

The young girl blossomed—that is, until Elizabeth's jealousy over her daughter's successes caused her to sabotage everything. Elizabeth would abruptly call her daughter home and accuse the host family of imaginary slights or ill intent. The host family had no official recourse because the girl hadn't *actually been placed in foster care. Repeatedly this happened, until, no matter what successes the progressively older girl experienced, she no longer believed that they would be lasting, and she began to sabotage her own efforts. The team that was ready to support mom and daughter never really could take shape because of Elizabeth's fear, jealousy, and lack of honesty, which caused pain for everyone involved.*

TOO MANY NEEDS

A care partner may have infinite needs, wants, or preferences. And while he should feel free to express these desires, you and the rest of the team may not be able to meet each and every one of them. And care partners will often have difficulty accepting that team members—who already feel pulled to make everything better—can't do *everything.* Together, though, the team should attempt to fulfill only the needs and wants that can be comfortably and reliably managed. You can devote your energy to identifying and finding resources from a broader personal safety net for the remaining tasks.

> Together, the team should attempt to fulfill only the needs and wants that can be comfortably and reliably managed.

Prioritizing needs is a skill that you will develop over time. As mentioned in Trisha's story in Chapter 4, one team we worked with prioritized their tasks this way: First, an action had to be *safe*. Then it needed to contribute to the care partner's *security*. Next, it had to be *simple*. And this safety, security, and simplicity had to lead to enhanced *serenity* for the care partner.

Using this team and its priorities as an example, you and your team can support one another in recognizing individual safety, security, simplicity, and serenity limits and preferences, too. One person may only be available mornings. Another might be willing to send e-mail messages or make phone calls. A third might organize meals or carpooling for kids. One might be best suited to accompany the care partner to doctor's appointments.

> Once you and your team have determined how to meet the most critical needs, you can seek community resources to tackle the other tasks.

Once you and your team have determined how to meet the most critical needs, you can seek community resources to tackle the other tasks. Consider contacting organizations that focus on seniors, single parents, various illnesses, or one of the many religious organizations and other entities that exist to meet needs in the community. You can find this information in the yellow pages, on the Internet, and through the organizations we've listed in the Resources section in the back of this book. You might also think of someone else to ask to join the team or brainstorm alternative strategies. Becoming familiar with these resources is another way to stretch your safety net.

MIX-UPS

Not everything goes perfectly smoothly. Even when your team appoints a leader or coordinator to assign specific times or tasks, a team member may just forget, drop the ball, or disappoint your care partner. Even if there are rosters and phone trees, and no one moves, loses a cell phone, or erases a database, there will still mostly likely be times when you forget something. This is just life.

> Be willing to laugh and keep things in perspective: This can be healing and leveling.

What can you do when someone "goofs" or miscommunicates? You could gently bring up the misunderstanding at a team meeting—not to assign blame, but to learn, improve, or make changes. Asking not "who was to blame" but rather "what factors contributed to this mix-up" is often useful in gathering data and preventing similar "goofs." Be willing to laugh and keep things in perspective: This can be healing and leveling.

Alternatively, if someone regularly drops her agreed-upon tasks, or if you follow a process that gets in the way rather than facilitates the care partner's health, assess what's going on and address it.

THE BOSSY PERSON

Some people view entering into a care-share team as their chance to "save" or "fix" the care partner or the situation. This is a typical response to wanting to help. Yet the entire team should remember that supporting, not fixing or saving, is the goal. Someone who wants to fix can tend to have specific ideas of how this should be done. But those "fixes" may not be what the care partner wants or needs—or even what the team can do. Group process can be a good balance for that, even if it is sometimes frustrating when it takes longer.

Being a member of a team has components of responsibility, while also demanding the relinquishing of control. A bossy person will be challenged to grow and behave more collaboratively as fellow team members become better at softly but firmly standing their ground. If someone becomes rude or starts bullying others, however, this is a different matter altogether: The group will need to work together to intervene— or perhaps this person herself needs to take a respite, seek counseling, or permanently leave the team. If the team member needs to leave, then, if possible, acknowledge whatever contributions she's made in the past as part of her leave taking.

A CRABBY CARE PARTNER

From time to time your care partner will probably feel emotional, fearful, or crabby. This may feel personal. It may be challenging. It may be too much.

Ben's Anger after His Stroke

Ben had always been independent and very clever at fixing things. After retiring from forty years as a Boeing engineer, Ben was happy to turn to the many home and hobby projects stored up for this time. He was totally caught off guard when he experienced a debilitating stroke. He felt cheated and robbed by the changes in his body. Ben eventually recovered most of his speech, as well as the use of his left arm and leg. However, he was a real challenge to be around due to his bitterness and anger. He would constantly lash out at others, and himself. Fortunately, as the months passed Ben slowly recovered and he became able to resume his projects and hobbies, and his bitterness and anger lessened. He even came to express some appreciation for the help his wife and other caregivers had offered. Without the team support, they added,

> *they'd have burnt out long before. In the end, team members could honestly say they were glad to have helped.*

One way to deflect a care partner's criticism and negativity is to prepare responses, such as "I hear how hard this is for you" or "I can only imagine how it seems from your perspective." Practice these before you need them. Get help in thinking up responses that are right for you.

Sometimes, though, whatever the situation it may be too much for you. When you're feeling overwhelmed, after making sure the care partner is safe, take a break and rejuvenate yourself: Walk around the block, call a team member for advice, take a soothing bath, do something artistic, or schedule time with a therapist or another person who is part of your own personal safety net. Do what you need to renew your sense of perspective. Don't let a crabby care partner drive you away from the chance to help and enrich your life.

> One way to deflect a care partner's criticism and negativity is to prepare responses. Practice these before you need them.

FEARS

It is perfectly normal and understandable to have some of your own fears, particularly when facing an illness, injury, or the unknown. Whether you are the person receiving care or someone who cares about that individual, fears will crop up. Naming them usually helps diminish their potency. Understanding your fears will help you avoid the kind of distancing behavior we've been addressing. Some fears that are fairly predictable are these:

> Whether you are the person receiving care or someone who cares about that individual, fears will crop up. Naming them usually helps diminish their potency.

Care Partner's Fears

- If I ask, will they say no?
- What will I do if they say yes?
- Will others be telling me what to do?
- If they help me now, how will I reciprocate? How can I ever pay them back?
- Will I lose control, privacy, or self-sufficiency?
- Will everyone know my problems?
- Will I need to go to an institution?

Team Member's Fears

- Will I be overwhelmed?

- Will I be able to do what's needed?

- What if she has a seizure or dies?

- What if I can't make things better?

- Will I have to do things that are too personal?

- What if I get sick, too?

In our experience as caregivers, we have heard people voice these fears—and successfully answer them, too. How *you* answer these questions will depend a lot on your unique history of experiences and your current circumstances. But we have found that saying them aloud or writing them down definitely helps.

Norma's Fear of Retirement Homes

Everyone who cared for Norma—her daughter, her son-in-law, two close women friends (who, like Norma, were also in their eighties), a home-health nurse, and a care manager counselor—agreed that Norma's memory problems and love of people could best be addressed in a retirement home. But they were stymied. Norma would visit lovely retirement homes, enjoy a meal there, chat with female residents, and seem to have a marvelous time. Yet at the last moment she would refuse to move. With time and sensitive conversations with a counselor, it became clear that Norma's reluctance stemmed from two deep fears. The first was historical: When Norma was eleven years old, her mother was placed in a tuberculosis sanatorium, which traumatized the whole family. She also feared that if she moved into a retirement home, she would forget how to do things, become old and dependent, and lose the love and respect of her family. Norma's team, despite heroic efforts, failed to allay these fears.

Norma did not move. Instead, her needs grew beyond what her care team could meet. Her safety net was not strong enough. She persisted in making unrealistic demands. Despite the best efforts of her small team, Norma's situation spun out of control, including many visits to the emergency room, police involvement, adult protective services, and attorneys.

Finally, it was determined that her risky, unrealistic, overly self-reliant behavior was a clear danger to herself. Still refusing to accept reasonable help, she had the right to self-determination taken from her and she was moved to a protective environment.

It's often true that when someone moves into a care facility, her world becomes smaller and smaller. The only information from the outside world may come through the television news, with its focus on crime, violence, and destruction. Even reading a newspaper may reinforce an isolated person's sense of powerlessness. This can cause distrust and anxiety. As Ram Dass said in the book *Still Here*, "When you shrink your world to your immediate surroundings, you end up trapped by them." How you respond to your care partner's fears and anxieties depends on circumstances, resources, and individuals. Clearly, though, compassion is called for—and again, humor. What are the fears and concerns? Can you help put words to them, even if they sound silly?

DEPRESSION

Grief is often confused with depression. And while the two states have much in common, there are some important differences. Grief is a normal response to an event or a situation experienced as a loss. Depression is an abnormal psychiatric disorder marked by persistent feelings of hopelessness and dejection, and sometimes by suicidal tendencies. Grief can lead to depression if unresolved. (Read more about grief in Chapter 8.)

If you suspect that someone you care about might be depressed, it's important to find out how to recognize depression.

Depression is a very serious condition and needs treatment. If you think you might be experiencing depression, seek help from a trained mental health specialist. Or if you suspect that someone you care about might be depressed, it's important to find out how to recognize depression. A good place to start is the following list compiled by the U.S. Department of Health and Human Services for older adults.

GUIDE TO RECOGNIZING DEPRESSION

When someone is depressed, that person has several symptoms nearly every day, all day, that last at least two weeks.

You can use the chart to check (x) off any symptoms you have had for two weeks or more.

☐ Loss of interest in things you used to enjoy, including sex *
☐ Feeling sad, blue, or down in the dumps *
☐ Feeling slowed down or restless and unable to sit still
☐ Feeling worthless or guilty
☐ Changes in appetite or weight loss or gain
☐ Thoughts of death or suicide; suicide attempts
☐ Problems concentrating, thinking, remembering, or making decisions
☐ Trouble sleeping or sleeping too much
☐ Loss of energy or feeling tired all of the time

Other symptoms include the following:

☐ Headaches
☐ Other aches and pains
☐ Digestive problems
☐ Sexual problems
☐ Feeling pessimistic or hopeless
☐ Being anxious or worried

If you have had five or more of these symptoms including at least one of the first two symptoms marked with an asterisk (*) for at least two weeks, you may have a major depressive disorder. See your health-care provider for diagnosis.

(U.S. Department of Health and Human Services, Public Health Service, *Depression Is a Treatable Illness: A Patient's Guide*, 1993)

LOSS OF CONTROL

In care-team relationships, as in any intense interpersonal experience, personality conflicts may arise. If your values and beliefs differ from your care partner's, this can cause friction. There are endless examples of how a care partner's and a team member's values may clash: Should you phone the doctor if the care partner shows signs of a slight fever and begins to cough, or only if he has difficulty breathing? Should the care partner dress himself, even if it's a laborious process? Should you inform the physician when the care partner exhibits new symptoms or honor his request to keep them "private"? Do you go ahead and install bars in the bathroom to

> As a team member, you may find yourself constantly weighing freedom versus safety, or honesty versus privacy.

prevent a care partner from falling, even when he hasn't requested them? As a team member, you may find yourself constantly weighing freedom versus safety, or honesty versus privacy.

In each of these scenarios, there's the possibility for the care partner to either maintain or lose control to some degree. There's also an opportunity for dialogue and increased understanding. It's important to remember that the care partner is the one who ultimately will live with the situation, and is the one who has the last word.

If, after discussion, you and another team member or your care partner still disagree, consider bringing the issue to the whole team to brainstorm a solution. Or seek the help of an experienced yet neutral third party, perhaps someone from Senior Services, a trusted family friend, or a trained counselor.

When making decisions that directly affect the care partner, carefully and compassionately think about all the areas in which she may be forced to give up control, especially if the issue is related to injury, illness, or advanced age: mobility, autonomy over simple daily tasks, privacy, personal appearance, bodily functions, and much more. It won't be easy for her to give up control, so tread delicately here; do the best you can to preserve her dignity.

> When making decisions that directly affect the care partner, carefully and compassionately think about all the areas in which she may be forced to give up control. Do the best you can to preserve her dignity.

If you're generally considered a "control freak," being a team member will be a great training ground for learning to let go. Even if you just want to oversee your *own* life, others may perceive you as overly controlling or bossy, though this may be far from your intention. Try to express your need for control by framing the issues broadly. Try to be curious about other ideas and possibilities. You control your own actions and reactions. You control how you define your needs. You cannot, however, exert control over anyone but yourself. Curiosity and compassion, once again, will be valuable tools.

Sharon and Rosie

Sharon was an African-American woman who had fought her way to success in her career. At forty years old, she was diagnosed with a terminal illness and given less than six months to live. But dying just wasn't on her radar screen. So she fought. She fought as she'd fought so many things in her life—and wouldn't admit that she had a disability or was dying. Still, it wasn't long before her doctors and family placed her in a Hospice setting.

Usually people who enter Hospice care say that they wish they'd done so earlier. But not Sharon. She continued to argue and fight, which made even running an errand for her or taking her to the park a difficult task. Friends and family found it hard to feel close to her and began to stay away. In the end, she had a hard fight and a lonely death.

Then there was Rosie. She, too, was African-American, successful, and under sixty. She had not expected her diagnosis, but received it with the grace with which she'd encountered much of life. The details of her illness, and her timeline, were similar to Sharon's, but Rosie's approach was to work with what came her way.

Rosie asked for help. She was going to find a way to take care of this task, too, as she'd taken care of so many, with love and dignity. She said that she was the only one in charge of the quality of her life. She would choose how and with whom to spend time, what to think about, what to pray for. Even in dying, Rosie chose well-being in every moment.

Within six weeks of her diagnosis, Rosie was dead. And though her death was no easier physically than Sharon's, for Rosie it came without argument or anger. Rosie died, as she had lived, with compassion for herself and others.

TOO MUCH HELP

Through our hands-on experience giving and sharing care, we have learned to identify many common "helping strategies" that actually complicate the situation or cause problems. Many of these attitudes and behaviors, while well-meaning, may cause a care partner to become weaker or more dependent upon you:

- Solving a problem for her because it's faster or easier for you to do it.
- Giving help before it is requested or without asking if it is wanted.
- Providing more care than is good for you, and thereby risking feeling overwhelmed or stressed.
- Not allowing her, if she wishes, the opportunity to try something where she may fail.
- Speaking for her.
- Needing her to need you.
- Not being honest about what you need or want.
- Overly protecting her from honest feedback about her words and actions.
- Trying to cover up or hide the reality of her situation.

In contrast, we have observed that when care-team members demonstrate the following attitudes and behaviors, they allow care receivers to develop and use their strength, flexibility, and resourcefulness.

- Openly and honestly communicating with the care partner.
- Clarifying roles, expectations, and limits.
- Communicating, negotiating, and partnering with him about what each will attempt to do.
- Being consistent and dependable, feeling responsible *to* but not *for* him.

- Doing your best to clarify assumptions and ask for feedback.
- Remembering to reach for humor and humility when other tools elude you.

Get Ready

Think:	*Can you separate being needy from asking for help?*
List:	*What scares you? List even the fears that sound silly.*
Get help:	*If you've seriously or specifically considered suicide, call 911 or your crisis center.*

CHAPTER 8
Prepare to Say Good-Bye

Few things last forever, including care-share teams and your participation in one. Acknowledging this reality from the start is a good step toward coping well when someone leaves the team, when the care partner gets better and no longer needs the team's help, or when the care partner dies. Some teams, originally centered on an illness or major life change, shift purpose and continue as some form of organized friendship. Most teams end, however, within a year. But many people find that, though the care team they've grown to love and appreciate may dissolve, they

> Some teams, originally centered on an illness or major life change, shift purpose and continue as some form of organized friendship.

can continue to share their compassion and use their new-found skills as part of yet another person's care-share team. People who have been helped often go on to help others. People who have helped once—and who have had a satisfying experience—often say yes to new opportunities.

Maria Lives

"I'm getting married!" gushed Maria. "He's the most handsome man I've ever met, he loves me to distraction, and why would we possibly want to wait? With both of our medical histories, this is the best time of our lives to commit. Will you stand up for me in our ceremony?"

Well, somewhere between elation for my friend and skepticism about the plan in general, I managed to say something supportive and even enthusiastic. Of course, I'd be there for her. I was a friend and one of her team members, wasn't I? Then I realized that a third part of my response was jealousy. I'd have to share her with someone else. My jealousy was followed by a sense of relief: I would share what sometimes felt like a burden. I struggled to balance all four reactions and emotions before finding equilibrium that felt comfortable.

Eight years before, Maria had received a heartbreaking diagnosis and was given six months to live. I had walked with Maria as she faced crisis after crisis, I had struggled to help her create positive ways to live her life as her capabilities decreased and medical issues mounted. I had varied my role in her caregiving with the changing scenarios, and I'd found ways to continue my commitment. Could I do it again this time? Did I want to?

I determined that I did want to stay in Maria's life. I sought professional counseling to sort it all out, and as I did, the answer became clear. I'd have to give up some of my role as best friend, confidant, and caregiver in favor of a simpler and more reciprocal friendship. Care-share team meetings— which once included eight or nine people—came down to only Maria, her case manager, and me. The meetings took a backseat to getting together for coffee and impromptu walks. It took some getting used to, but this was the beginning of a sweet time for Maria, her new husband, and me. After all, Maria had gotten stronger. She was capable of more flexibility and mutuality. And though her illness had progressed, she'd simultaneously grown healthier—focusing less on lesions and more on the world outside of her. As for me, I'd had to give up being the one who always gave. And until the day when Maria may again need more from me, I'll enjoy this freedom and the expanded friendship it's allowed.

ENDINGS AND BEGINNINGS

Lives change, and every change involves both a beginning and an ending. Not all persons who think they will be able to participate can do so, and not all can do so for the life of the team. It's important to value all that transpired and all the effort put forth no matter the outcome—whether a care partner recovers or dies, or whether a team member chooses to leave or is fired. Sometimes the current reality causes us to want to rewrite history to either sanitize or satirize the situation. But as Will Rogers said, "Never let yesterday use up too much of today." Once you've acknowledged, respected, and let go of the past, it's important to move on. Talk with other team members about honoring each other's contributions as you go along and marking departures as they happen. It's important to say good-bye, to take time for some sort of ritual, and to allow emotional space for grieving—even if the changes are "for the good."

> It's important to say good-bye, to take time for some sort of ritual, and to allow emotional space for grieving—even if the changes are "for the good."

Reinhold Niebuhr has said, with great wisdom: "Give me the serenity to accept what cannot be changed. Give me the courage to change what can be changed. And give me the wisdom to know one from the other." You can be certain that change will come. You know you can't control it. Thinking through how you'll acknowledge the past and address the future will help you maintain a positive balance and attitude.

Large or small, losses are often accompanied by strong emotions that may challenge your emotional stability and your sense of self, whether you are the care partner or a care-team member walking beside him. In the following story, John tells of his journey with Deborah, whose good-bye rituals eased her losses.

Deborah's Many Good-Byes

The human resources director at her company initially requested my professional assistance in Deborah's case. She was a professional in her late forties who had early-onset Alzheimer's-type dementia and could no longer function in her important capacity at her firm.

Because Deborah had no living relatives but many friends, I suggested to the human resources director that we help Deborah create a care-share team. She agreed and hired me to set up and mentor the team of friends and co-workers, who worked together for what ended up being a five-year journey.

Deborah's close friend and colleague stepped up to serve as team coordinator. This heroic friend, along with other team members, bravely walked with Deborah as Alzheimer's gradually erased her knowledge, memories, and many skills and abilities.

For Deborah, there were many good-byes: First, her job. Her colleagues donated sick days and vacation time as a gift to

Deborah. They invited her to lunch during those weeks when she no longer "worked" but still "dropped by." They hosted a big party to mark her "early retirement" (as they chose to call it).

In the next three months, she said good-bye to her car and her driver's license. She reluctantly gave up paying her bills and managing her health-care appointments, and eventually moved out of her home. Each of these good-byes was accompanied by another ritual to help her grieve what she must leave behind and hand off to her team the tasks that would lighten her load.

Next came the need for twenty-four-hour supervision and a move into an assisted living home. That's where her care team hosted a final party in her honor. When Deborah lost her ability to recognize most of the members of her team, most felt it was more than they could bear and withdrew from the team.

Deborah's last move was into a nursing home, where a structured and protective environment and caring, specialized staff safeguarded her. Only a couple of team members, the nursing home staff, and I supported the remainder of Deborah's journey.

Deborah's story is both heartbreaking and encouraging. Although her team members were saddened by Deborah's losses, they also were forever changed by the enriching experience, the camaraderie, the knowledge of the difference they made, and what they learned about themselves and the other members of the team. Creating and participating in rituals to ease her transitions also helped all of them become more aware of their own emotions. Looking forward to what was next helped them discover the positive aspects of walking through a difficult passage. Several people later told us stories of other teams they helped form thereafter. You've read some of those stories.

> Having a ritual of sorts for saying good-bye to team members who are leaving honors their good work and commitment, as well as the relationship you've formed with them.

Another kind of gift was bestowed unknowingly to a friend, who tells the next story. The gift came through Martha's ability, even as she was dying, to remain curious about new ideas—and to then let her friend know that an idea had taken hold.

Martha's Gift to Her Friends

The greatest gift I received from Martha came about a month before she died. In a phone message, she acknowledged that she never would have believed that what I had once said could be true in her life. During the course of her illness, she'd been profoundly uncomfortable with friends coming together. Yet an unexpected event caused her to reconsider. Two friends had accidentally come to visit her in the hospital at the same time. They met at her bedside, and as they were chatting they discovered a common bond: Both of their daughters were soon going off to college. The surprise for me was Martha's acknowledging delight in hearing them chat about this shared wonder and challenge. I like to think that her final days were eased knowing that her friends had one another. It was, at last, not just a collection of friends, but a team.

SAYING GOOD-BYE TO TEAM MEMBERS

Good-bye rituals are not only important for care partners, but they're also helpful for team members. Having a ritual of sorts for saying good-bye to team members who are leaving honors their good work and commitment, as well as the relationship you've formed with them. The idea is to arrange a formal good-bye for the one who is leaving regardless of the circumstances of their departure, whether it's an out-of-town move, a schedule conflict, or a health crisis.

Vivian Needed to End Care-Sharing Team Membership

Vivian had been a member of the care-sharing team helping

Joan care for her husband, Wayne, who had Alzheimer's. As Wayne's dementia grew worse, caring for him was beginning to remind Vivian of her dark, lonely days caring for her father. She realized she needed more time to heal from the long, hard journey of her dad's illness. She wanted to help her dear friends Wayne and Joan, but knew in her heart she couldn't continue as part of the team.

Joan had anticipated that some friends and family members would eventually drop out, so she had recruited an extra large care-sharing team. When Vivian spoke of her need to leave, Joan gathered this team together and suggested hosting a potluck party to celebrate and thank her friend. Vivian at first refused, saying she felt like a quitter and didn't deserve a party. But Joan reminded Vivian that she had already contributed an important, lasting gift—and for that Joan would be forever grateful.

At Joan's request, I, her pastor, retold one of Mother Theresa's stories. Mother Theresa was originally partnered with another sister who was scheduled to travel to India with her, but at the last moment the sister suffered a health crisis and could not go. This sister, however, agreed to be Mother Theresa's "spiritual partner." And while she could not give hands-on care, she could still be of great value to Mother Theresa. Joan asked Vivian if she would pray for her and be her "spiritual partner." Vivian, through tearful eyes, agreed, gave *up her guilt feelings, and went on to enjoy the rest of the celebration—her celebration—as her hands-on caregiving for Wayne ended and her spiritual support of Joan began.*

LEAVING UNDER ROCKY CIRCUMSTANCES

Some family conflicts or personal styles may so offend a team member that he or she quits in anger. If care-team members feel they can no longer support the situation, then leaving the group is the most responsible decision.

Care Team Disaster

They both believed their mom needed more help than they could provide and set about asking for help. Unfortunately, they couldn't agree on what was needed and who should provide it. And as is sometimes the case with sisters, they were competitive with each other. One of the ways this came out was in each one questioning what the other sister did for their mother. They also disagreed over their mom's level of functioning, how compromised her memory was, and if she was depressed. Professional health-care providers, friends, and other family who wanted and tried to help were frustrated by the conflicting messages and requests. Several paid in-home caregivers finally quit. A couple of friends stopped helping. In time, fewer and fewer people were willing to deal with the frustrations and misunderstandings that the sisters created. Both they and their mother suffered.

Care-team members should prepare for the possibility that the care partner may fire one or several of them, due to personality conflicts, differences in opinions, unprofessional conduct, or concerns regarding reliability. Whatever the reason, whether it seems fair or not, the care partner has the right to do this. If it becomes necessary to say good-bye, developing and following a protocol for leave taking will be helpful.

> If it becomes necessary to say good-bye, developing and following a protocol for leave taking will be helpful.

WHEN THE CARE PARTNER RECOVERS

Good-byes may also be necessary if your care partner gets well, and the care-share team is no longer needed in its current form. This was true for Maria in the first story of this chapter, as well as for Martin in the story below.

Martin Comes Full Circle

When Martin came to Seattle he was ill, alone, and tired. He joined a church that matched him with a faith-based group of individuals who welcomed Martin as their care partner, supplying him with weekly dinners, occasional movie and popcorn nights, and a lot of listening. Over several months, Martin came to trust this group of newfound friends. He came out of his shell enough to confide in them. He was surprised when they became closer, rather than draw away or try to change him.

Martin's health began to improve as he settled into a more stable life, took his medications regularly, ate, and began to have the energy to exercise a little. He began to express his gratitude to his team for their generosity. Then, one week he surprised his care-share team members by cooking dinner for them.

A while later, Martin surprised everyone again when he joined a team that would support someone else who needed a safety net. He said this was his opportunity to pay forward all the goodness he had received. Martin had come full circle.

WHEN THE CARE PARTNER DIES

When someone close to you passes on, you'll most likely move through a range of feelings. You may ponder the awe, wonder, and mystery of life. You may feel angry or unsettled as you're reminded that life is fragile, and precious. It does indeed, at just one moment in time, stop. The suddenness and decisiveness of the moment of death may leave you feeling powerless. Even thoughtful preparation is likely to leave you surprised or touched in unexpected ways.

Good-Bye Dad: I Love You

David and I, his counselor, had talked a great deal about what it might be like if he were with his dad when his dad passed on. David had believed he was psychologically prepared, but now he wasn't so sure. His father's breathing was slow, loud, and raspy, and his eyes didn't appear to be seeing anything.

David realized that his own breathing was synchronized with his dad's. "We've always been close," David thought. Tears welled up in his eyes as, once again, a wave of sadness washed over him. He reached over onto the bed where his father lay and took his hand. It felt weak and bony and frail but David was, nonetheless, glad to hold it. He was thankful for these past few days with his father and, in a way that surprised him, for the opportunity to touch his dad and hold his hand. While a loving family, they had not been very physical in their display of caring. David sat quietly for a moment as thoughts of growing up and years past swept through his mind.

Suddenly, pulled back from his reflections, David realized his father had silently, gently passed on. Tears streamed down his cheeks as he sat marveling at the mystery of life. David waited a few minutes longer, still holding his father's hand, and let memories and feeling float past. Finally, once again with gratitude for all his father and family had shared, David squeezed his father's hand for the last time and whispered, "Good-bye Dad, I love you."

It may also be that, though you are prepared for the death, there are other surprises waiting as funeral arrangements and rituals of leave taking arise.

Sam's Story: A Clash of Cultures and Rituals

Sam had developed dementia in his late fifties, which was not uncommon for someone born with Down's syndrome. His frail, elderly parents visited almost daily whenever health permitted, but two years earlier they had entrusted his full-time care to the staff of an adult family home. Sam's good nature had quickly won the hearts of the staff despite his limited use of language. The staff members themselves came from five different countries and spoke limited English.

When Sam died, the staff needed a "debriefing" because of their cultural diversity and differing attitudes toward and rituals around death. One staff member reported that in her culture it was a deep honor and show of love to bathe and carefully dress the person who had just passed on. Another warned that, in her culture, only family members could be allowed to look at the deceased person. Another staff member commented that no one was to touch or move the deceased until a spiritual person or a person of God had been allowed to help the spirit leave the body. Another staff person, one who had resided in this country longer, felt strongly that no one should act until the family of the deceased arrived to make a decision.

Despite—perhaps even because of—the fact that Sam's caregivers came from different cultures and held diverse views of death, Sam's story still had a good ending. Sam's parents came in to make the needed decisions and with sensitivity reassured the staff that all was okay. They invited the staff to join them in a celebration of Sam's life and explained that this was part of their family's practice. Everyone agreed to do so.

Sometimes the care partner knows that death is near. When a person expresses that he is ready to go, as Carl did in the story below, saying good-bye may be comfortable and the passing easy. His daughter, Pastor Catherine Fransson, tells this story in what she called a "spirit stone."

Rest in Peace

His desk calendar was at Monday, August 8. On Wednesday the 10th, the nursing staff administered a small dose of morphine to allay his growing anxiety. Hospice had been agreed to, but he had met only one or two of their staff. Thursday when he walked fully dressed, walker-in-hand, to his shower, he told the aide, Debbie, he was dying. She told him she loved him, and he said I love you, too. They hugged. And at 2 a.m. on Friday, August 12, they found him in his small bed, still, his face calm. No extraordinary measures were ordered.

Five weeks after his 101st birthday, Carl Abner stepped out of this dimension and embarked on a new adventure.

I meet the nurses who saw Dad through. I hear the stories of his final hours and days. There are tears in their eyes as well as mine; they cared for him, loved him over the three and a half years this was his home: a good home, a place of caring and respect, of enough space for the way he needed to live his life, and of not a little joy.

Who would have thought my father's move to a nursing home would become such a gift in so many ways? His relinquishing the authority he'd wielded all his life. His relaxing into the routine. His comfort at being left alone. The freedom to do whatever he chose within the constraints of the place. He read the Wilson Quarterly, two newspapers, two *news magazines, and the dictionary, always delighted to discover new meanings.*

Here I discovered his deep shyness, his inability to hold two ideas in juxtaposition, his inability to imagine another scenario from the reality he experienced; and his great loyalty to my mother, his deep faith, his graciousness for all those who helped him through the day, and his gratefulness for my own regular weekly appearance at his side, listening, responding, asking questions, and—may I be frank?—getting acquainted.

His pastor once said of him, I have never met such a Lutheran conscience. I am not sure what that means, but I think it's a left-handed compliment. Maybe that's all the compliment any of us gets: an admiring on-looker, envious of the iron will, the constitution, and the sense of humor that gets any of us from 1904 to 2005, or 1942 to 2043, when I will reach his age.

My dad will rest in peace; he would have nothing less.

– Blessings from Catherine Fransson, August 19, 2005

In contrast to Carl Abner's story, in Ginny's case, all agreed that she died "before her time." The team members all knew months in advance that she was dying, and individually and collectively they had dealt with the anger, unfairness, and diverse other feelings that arise when a young person dies. Thus, having done this emotional work toward acceptance, the team was better able to celebrate the joy of Ginny's life at her memorial service.

A Celebration of Ginny's Life

Ginny was a brilliant scholar who, at age thirty-eight, developed a cancer in her brain. For eleven months, friends and family formed a close care-share team and partnered with Hospice to help Ginny pass on amid love and care.

The ceremony was held in a small interdenominational church. Pictures of Ginny surrounded the pews. All who attended, including the care-share team members, had been invited to bring memories to share. During the three-hour service, there was much grieving, crying, a lot of laughter, and joy as memories were shared. The care-team members were so touched by the ceremony that they decided to gather one year later to again celebrate Ginny's life.

GRIEF 101

A Cut Finger

Is numb before it bleeds,
t bleeds before it hurts,
It hurts until it begins to heal,
It forms a scab and itches until finally, the scab is gone
And a small scar is left where once there was a wound.

Grief is the deepest wound you have ever had.

Like a cut finger, it goes through stages and leaves a scar.

– Author Unknown

Care partners may grieve at different times—and in different ways—than their care team. Being part of a care team gives you multiple opportunities to become knowledgeable about grief and to become a good griever. In small and large ways, life demands that we grieve our losses, harvest our memories, and move on. Even "positive" changes—a new job, a move, a

As you learn to recognize complex emotions, you will become better prepared for the time when you encounter a huge loss.

marriage, a birth—involve losses. The old job, the house left behind, a more complex or a more carefree life are gone. The euphoria of the positive is often balanced with an unrecognized sense of loss. With this may come confusion. Simply noticing this will help you manage that emotion. What's more, there are many valuable books, articles, Web sites, grief counselors, and other resources focusing on understanding, experiencing, and eventually passing through grief. As you learn to recognize complex emotions, you will become better prepared for the time when you encounter a huge loss.

Ezra Makes Peace with His Grief and Anger

Ezra told me he had been born in the Midwest into a family with nothing. Through extreme hard work and self-sacrifice they become moderately successful. Unfortunately for young Ezra, there was far too little time and attention for this sensitive and intellectually gifted boy. Additionally, his father, who was raised in Europe during very difficult times, was harsh in word and action with Ezra.

As his father aged, Ezra was forced into a caregiving role for this frail and difficult man. In my consulting and counseling with Ezra, a complex picture emerged. Ezra felt a deep mixture of anger and grief over all he had missed, over some of the ways he had been treated, and over what he had hoped to receive from his father before he died. As he sorted out these emotions and fully experienced his feelings, Ezra slowly came to make peace with it all and found that his caregiving time with his difficult father became a little easier. Ezra also discovered meaning and significance in the many ways he had been different from his father in parenting his own two sons. Ezra also reported feeling more open and expressive with family and friends.

The "up-close time" that illness brings can give you a new awareness and understandings of yourself and others. Both healing and renewed growth can be a valuable part of your journey forward.

Everything in this life comes to an end. Even when the care team you form ends, you can expand your understanding of complex emotions. Consider the following:

- You quit the care-share team, perhaps because you can no longer commit the time, you move, or you are burnt out. You likely will feel relief, guilt, fear for the care partner, or adrift from the team, who've supported you emotionally.

- The care partner dies, and the team dissolves or decides to meet annually to commemorate the passing. You may feel grief, anger, or gratitude for the time you spent helping and for the camaraderie of the team.

- The care partner gets better and no longer needs help. You may feel glad for the care partner, but sad to say good-bye to the team. You may feel equally happy you no longer have to deal with team complexities.

- The care partner dismisses everyone, and you experience anger and relief.

Whatever the reason for the team ending, you likely will experience complex feelings: relief mixed with sorrow, anger combined with guilt, or fear overlaid with depression. All of this is normal and needs to be accepted, experienced, understood, and passed through to the other side. What's important to remember is that with loss comes grief. Grieving is necessary for healing and moving on.

THE GRIEF PROCESS

When the team ends, especially when the care partner dies, each member of the team will experience some form of grief. To resolve and move through your grief, it's helpful to understand Elizabeth Kubler-Ross's spiral grief model. Unresolved grief comes from trying to jump from one side of the cycle to the other without acknowledging and experiencing all of your feelings. Not everyone will experience these feelings in the same order, but most people experience most of these emotions at some point during loss and change. Typically, the emotions come and go.

> Whatever the reason for the team ending, you likely will experience complex feelings: relief mixed with sorrow, anger combined with guilt, or fear overlaid with depression. All of this is normal and needs to be accepted, experienced, understood, and passed through to the other side.

Especially for some men, the grief process may be quite difficult, often because it is denied. Most men have learned from a very early age to control and often hide or suppress their feelings. Men often learn these lessons so well that they develop deep, usually no longer conscious, habits of not showing or not even feeling their sorrow, fear, and loneliness. Interestingly, we have observed that sometime around age fifty, men lose the ability to "rise above" or "sidestep" these feelings and must relearn how to grieve, to experience the feelings Kubler-Ross describes. This actually helps them to eventually heal and move on.

There are many ways we experience grief. Grief can show up as fear, anger, or emotional withdrawal. Some people have a way of shedding tears internally without showing a single drop on the outside. Thus, many of us must counter strong anti-grieving learning while trying to learn how to grieve and mourn. We urge you to get to know your ways of grieving, to learn to grieve, and to let grief pass through you as do the other emotions.

Gifted grief counselor Bonnie Genevay has compiled this list of "ways of grieving" to help people begin to make a space for, or practice, grieving:

- Writing (journal, diary, poetry, letter to a friend, or letter to the lost one).
- Talking about the loss, expressing feelings (with a friend, with a family member, in a grief support group, with a counselor).

- Walking (allowing nature to bring forth memories, feelings); running.
- Sitting with a person who knows of your grief, not talking but sharing the silence.
- Crying; joining others as they cry.
- Slowing down in behavior and thought so that the meaning of the loss can surface and you can understand the depth of loss.
- Raging; allowing the anger inherent in grief to emerge through words or the voice (i.e., cussing in your car on the freeway).
- Touching (holding hands, holding someone else who shares the grief, hugging/being hugged all elicit feelings of grief).
- Throwing rocks in a stream.
- Listening to music.
- Painting, drawing, creating art.

CYCLES OF LOSS

It's strange that anyone could make any sense out of the confusing and changing constellation of feelings, thoughts, actions, physical sensations, and social changes that can accompany losses of those we love. But there are common characteristics that have been identified, most notably by Elizabeth Kubler-Ross.

From the time of the loss, you will cycle through shock, denial, anger, and guilt; bargaining, fear, and tears; despair and depression; and resignation, adjustment, and acceptance before reaching a point that can be called recovery. You may find yourself frequently returning several times (and in no predictable order) to steps you've visited before. Not everyone will experience all of these steps, and they won't come in predictable order. The above list is very general, but has been tested and is generally true. Trying to jump from loss to recovery without acknowledging feelings or taking time for them frequently results in unresolved and complicated grief reactions, frequently leading to depression.

The cycle of loss never truly closes, because experiencing the loss and its grief changes you forever. How you are changed depends on your own attitude and determination. New depth of character and strength may emerge. Bitterness, anger, and withdrawal are the other end of a spectrum, with many variations in between.

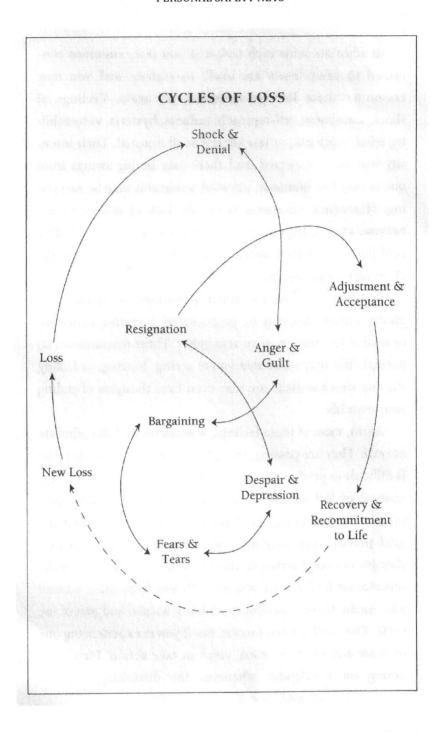

CYCLES OF LOSS

Shock &
Denial

Adjustment &
Acceptance

Resignation

Anger &
Guilt

Loss

Bargaining

New Loss

Despair &
Depression

Recovery &
Recommitment
to Life

Fears &
Tears

In addition, with each new loss you face, emotions connected to prior losses are likely to surface, and you may encounter these leftover emotions yet again. Feelings of shock, numbness, self-reproach, sadness, hysteria, vulnerability, relief, craziness, or fear are not at all unusual. Their intensity may be unexpected, and there may be big swings from one to another. Similarly, physical sensations may be surprising. Headaches, shortness of breath, lack of energy, excess nervous energy, hypersensitivity to noise, dry mouth, hot or cold flashes, stomach upsets, clumsiness, or tightness in the chest may come and go.

At times, you may encounter sensations that seem completely unreal. You may be preoccupied, forgetful, confused, or unable to concentrate or remember. These reactions are all normal. You may sense that you're seeing, hearing, or feeling the one who has died; you may even have thoughts of ending your own life.

Again, most of these feelings, sensations, and thoughts are normal. They are passing, though the length of time they last is difficult to predict. You may suffer recurring bouts of sleeplessness or feel absent-minded. At times, you may seek solitude or want the company of others. As you move through the grief process, you may also experience changes in dreams, changes in sexual activities, marital difficulties, anxiety, or the unwelcome feeling that you are different from those around you. Again, these experiences are normal and part of the cycle. They will not last forever, but if you're experiencing one or more and are concerned, you can act. First, note on a calendar whenever the disturbing thought, feeling, or action occurs. Track this over, say, three months. This will provide valuable input. Next, you could keep a journal, which will give you the same kind of data as the calendar, with more emotional detail. Or seek professional counseling. Our experience tells us that the first two steps often eliminate the need for the third. (While a fleeting thought of ending your life is normal, if you find yourself seriously considering ending your life, please call a crisis hot line for help.)

If you can treat yourself gently, stay with the feelings a little while, and trust that you are not alone in feeling this way; these unusual intruders will soften and diminish.

If, however, you can treat yourself gently, stay with the feelings a little while, and trust that you are not alone in feeling this way (people over the millennia have encountered the same grief process), these unusual intruders will soften and diminish. "I can't stand it" may slowly become "I'm prepared to move on."

HELPING SOMEONE WHO IS GRIEVING

If you know someone who is grieving, you may worry about saying or doing the wrong thing. When you are thinking about what to say to someone who is facing a loss, reflect upon your own grief experiences—what words and actions comforted you? Here are a few simple suggestions from people in grief about expressions that were helpful and those that were hurtful.

THINGS THAT HURT

- Being avoided: People didn't know what to say or do; they avoided talking with me. They were uncomfortable, but it made me feel isolated.

- Being pushed to talk: Sometimes I didn't feel like talking, and sometimes people were nosey and kept asking what was wrong. A gentle knock at the door is what I welcomed—then, I could talk, or not.

- Being told how to feel: I was told I should cry or I shouldn't cry. I shouldn't be angry. I should feel better by now. People assume I should feel a certain way because "everyone feels that way." My feelings are my own, not right or wrong, they are just what I feel. There are no rules for grieving.

THINGS THAT HELPED

- What meant the most was knowing that people were thinking of me and that they cared.

- Helping others: When I helped other people, it made me feel better. It took my attention away from my grief.

- Talking: When I felt like talking, I was grateful to friends who weren't afraid to listen and share.

- Laughing: I also learned that it wasn't wrong to laugh and have a good time. Laughing gave me the same kind of relief that crying did.

- Hugging/affection: A hug from a friend often made me happier that any words a friend could say.

- Being with friends: I liked it when my friends asked me to do things with them in the same old normal ways. I liked it when they came to the house and also when they took me away from the house.

We've included the lists above to help you think about how to comfort a grieving person and how to be more at home with personal grief. Grief can indeed "wash us larger," that is, deep experiences can leave us with greater inner and relational capacities. Being reminded of this fragility and passing nature of life—cherishing what has been and savoring what's ahead—are gifts that, though difficult and uncomfortable, have value.

CHILDREN GRIEVE, TOO

While an in-depth discussion is beyond the scope of this book, we must point out that children grieve, too. Many excellent resources are listed in the Bibliography and Resources sections in the back of the book. Whether a child is ill, exposed to divorce, or missing the time and attention that must now be given to addressing significant life changes, he will need to express his grief. Care-share teams can include older children in the care plan to help fill the gaps left by a parent or sibling who is ill or emotionally unavailable. What's more, one of the many joys that may come from team participation is spending time with a child and playing an important role in her ongoing growth and development. She benefits by participating—and so does the rest of the team.

Grieving is a child's normal and healthy response when someone in his or her life is ill, is no longer the same, or has changed. Every child has an innate ability to heal. Like an adult, each child grieves in her own unique way. The way to assist a child's grieving process is to give truthful information, listen carefully, and provide acceptance, caring, and a lot of love.

Marking endings and losses as well as beginnings, through ritual and ceremony, is an opportunity for the community to come together, share, and grow more solid and to note and celebrate what has been done. We've just scratched the surface of this important topic and urge you to learn all you can about how to survive and even thrive during life's inevitable losses and endings.

GET READY

Talk with the group: What will you do if someone decides to leave?

Pay attention: What are the little things that the care partner is losing?

Think: How do you deal with good-byes and endings? What do you need to do to be better prepared? Do it.

Conclusion

We feel stronger and safer because of our own personal safety nets. Having taken opportunities to prepare, we've pulled safety nets together, taken control of changes and challenges, created care-share teams, and been supported in ways that have surprised and enriched us.

Believe in the power and strength of taking control during changing, challenging, and uncertain times.

We hope that you, too, have come to believe in the power and strength of taking control during changing, challenging, and uncertain times. We've selected the stories as examples of the many inspiring people and events we've encountered. We think they show the personal courage and flexibility that can surface in recognizing a desire for help and asking for it.

We hope we've demonstrated that it is a real gift to yourself and your loved ones when you bring this courage and honesty forward.

Are you now ready to create your own safety net? Or to strengthen the one you have? We hope so.

Are you now more prepared to be a member of a care-share team? Do you have a better sense of what one can do? Do you have a vision of what the beginning, middle, and end of a care-share team might look like?

Do you feel more personal flexibility and freedom to participate in ways that both work for you and still contribute to the care-share team? We hope so.

If you're starting to develop an image of our communities covered by interlocking and overlapping networks of safety nets, then once again we have been successful. We see a world covered by large and small connecting and overlapping safety nets. We are buoyed, inspired, and made bolder by this image—and hope you are, too.

- Take Control.
- Get Ready.
- Get Connected.

Bibliography

Albom, Mitch. *Tuesdays with Morrie.* New York: Broadway Books, 1997.

The main character, Morrie, suffering from ALS, explores care receiving and living life fully.

Alzheimer's Disease and Related Disorders Newsletter. Chicago: Alzheimer's Disease and Related Disorders Association.

For a copy of this newsletter, contact the national association at 800-621-0379 or your local Alzheimer's chapter.

Armstrong, Lance, and Sally Jenkins. *It's Not About the Bike: My Journey Back to Life.* New York: Berkley Books, 2000.

This is Lance Armstrong's story of his battle with cancer, his "support team," and a bit about his life as a bicycle racer.

Babcock, Elise NeeDell. When Life Becomes Precious: The Essential Guide for Patients, Loved Ones, and Friends of Those Facing Serious Illnesses. New York: Bantam Books, 1997.

This guide contains hundreds of tips for helping patients and caregivers deal with cancer.

Barg, Gary. The Fearless Caregiver: How to Get the Best Care for Your Loved One and Still Have a Life of Your Own. Sterling, VA: Capital, 2003.

Barg defines a family member's role in developing a care plan for a loved one in today's health care system.

Bolen, Jean Shinoda. *Close to the Bone.* New York: Touchstone, 1996.

This therapist tells of women battling cancer and their support systems through the lens of Jungian theory and mythology.

Carter, Rosalynn, and Susan MaGolant. *Helping Yourself Help Others: A Book for Caregivers.* New York: Times Books, 1996.

The authors identify strategies, support groups, programs, organizations, and books to assist caregivers of the elderly and mentally ill.

Coposselo, Cappy, and Sheila Warnock. *Share the Care.* New York: Simon & Schuster, 2004.

This guide is useful for creating a "caregiver family" to meet the daily challenges of providing care, especially focusing on cancer.

Cughlan, Patricia. *Facing Alzheimer's: Family Caregivers Speak.* New York: Ballantine Books, 1993.

    Cughlan describes the personal experiences of many families.

Dass, Ram. Still Here: Embracing Aging, Changing and Dying. New York: Riverhead Books, 2000.

    A psychological guru describes his life and the life-changing and enhancing wisdom he encountered after his stroke.

Duda, Deborah. *Coming Home.* Santa Fe, NM: John Muir Publications, 1984.

    This is a guide to dying at home with dignity.

Fransson, Catherine. E-mail to "Spirit Stones" mailing list, Number 148, August 2005.

    This is Pastor Fransson's last essay in a series of reflections she wrote while caring for her parents in their final days of life.

Garfield, Charles, Cindy Spring, and Sedonia Cahill. *Wisdom Circles: A Guide to Self-Discovery and Community Building in Small Groups.* New York: Hyperion, 1998.

Gibson, John, and Bonnie Brown Hartley. *The Dynamics of Aging Families: A Handbook for Adult Children.* Venice, FL: Cambio Press, 2006.

The authors give practical explanations and hypothetical scenarios of family dynamics for adult children and aging parents, with one half of the book written for adult children and one half written for their aging parents.

Gibson, John, and Bonnie Brown Hartley. *Health-Care Issues of Aging Families: A Handbook for Adult Children.* Venice, FL: Cambio Press, 2006.

The authors give practical explanations and hypothetical scenarios for adult children and aging parents on how to be prepared for changing health, with one half of the book written for adult children and one half written for their aging parents.

Hintz Fordyce, Christine, Elizabeth N. Oettinger, and Dennis E. Kenny. *Aging in Stride.* Seattle: Caresource Healthcare Communications, Inc., 2004.

This excellent resource is a thorough guide for older adults.

Hooyman, Nancy, and Wendy Lustbader. *Taking Care of Your Aging Family Members: A Practical Guide.* New York: Free Press, 1994.

The authors give practical, sensitive, and expert guidance that will help in dealing with myriad issues of aging family members.

How to Hire Helpers: A Guide for Elders and Their Families. Seattle: The Church Council of Greater Seattle, Taskforce on Aging.

This excellent brochure about health-care decisions for aging adults and their families is available by calling 206-525-1213.

Hughes, Pat M. *Gracious Space*. Seattle: Center for Ethical Leadership, 2004.

Hughes has written a delightful little book about creating space in our lives, relationships, and world.

James, John W., and Frank Cherry. *The Grief Recovery Handbook: A Step-by-Step Program for Moving Beyond Loss*. New York: Harper & Row Publishers, 1988.

The authors have developed a practical and sensitive guidebook.

Kenny, Dennis E., and Elizabeth N. Oettinger, editors. The Family Care Book: A Comprehensive Guide for Families of Older Adults, 1991.

This award-winning resource is independently published and available from http://www.caresource.com.

Living. A newsletter published by Providence Mount Saint Vincent (the Mount), 4831 35th Ave SW, Seattle, WA 98126-2779; 206-937-3700; http://www.providence.org.

Lowe, Elizabeth. Care Pooling: How to Get the Help You Need to Care for the Ones You Love.San Francisco: Berrett-Koehler Publishers, 1993.

Lowe has written a practical guide to organizing help for both everyday and extraordinary caregiving.

Lundberg, Gary, and Joy Lundberg. *I Don't Have to Make Everything All Better.*New York: Viking Press, 1999.

Learn to improve one-to-one communication in a variety of situations.

Lustbader, Wendy. *Counting on Kindness: The Dilemmas of Dependency.* New York: The Free Press, 1991.

This is an excellent book about feelings for both caregivers and especially care receivers.

Mace, Nancy L., and Peter V. Rabins. *The 36-Hour Day.* Baltimore: Johns Hopkins University Press, 1991.

This practical and helpful guide is for caregivers of relatives with some form of dementia.

Massie, Lynne. I'll Be Here Tomorrow: Transforming Tragedy into Triumph. Tumwater, WA: Cymitar Press, 2004.

Just what the title says.

Menten, Ted. Gentle Closings: How to Say Good-Bye to Someone You Love. Philadelphia: Running Press, 1991.

Menten guides the reader through coping with the loss of a loved one, exploring survivor guilt issues, and stages of grief.

Miller, D. Patrick. A Little Book of Forgiveness: Challenges and Meditations for Anyone with Something to Forgive. Berkeley: Fearless Books, 1994.

Monroe, Peggy, with Judy Gough and Tim Grendon. *Circles of Care.* Seattle, WA: AIDS Caregiver Support Network, 1998.

This well-focused guide is for those who want to support AIDS patients.

Morris, Virginia. *How to Care for Aging Parents: A Complete Guide.* New York: Workman Publishing, 1996.

This is a smart, compassionate, timely book for anyone with aging family members.

Mundy, Michaelene. Sad Isn't Bad: A Good-Grief Guidebook for Kids Dealing with Loss. St. Meinrad, IN: Abbey Press, 1998.

Nesmith, Alison. *When You Care: Perspectives from 15 Years of Care Sharing.* Bellevue, WA: Overlake Hospital Medical Center, 2003.

Oliver, Mary. *Long Life: Essays and Other Writings*. Cambridge, MA: Da Capo Press, 2004.

Oliver selects personal essays and other writings related to her observations and experiences with growing older.

Porter-O'Grady, Tim, and Cathleen Krueger Wilson. *The Health Care Teambook*. St. Louis, MO: Mosby, 1998.

This book informs, engages, and invites care professionals to participate in team work for the benefit of aging parents—and themselves.

Resnick, Barbara. Restorative Care Nursing for Older Adults: A Guide for All Care Settings. New York: Springer Publishing Center, 2004.

The author describes the tools needed to establish a restorative care program. This presents a philosophical basis, rather than a plan.

Romney, Rodney. "Making Friends with Our Own Death." May 17, 2005. http://www.writersden.com/rodneyromney.

The Rev. Dr. Rodney Romney, now retired, was an American Baptist pastor for 40 years, most recently at Seattle First Baptist Church.

Royer, Ariela. *Life with Chronic Illness*. Westport, CT: Praeger Publishers, 1998.

The author explores social and psychological dimensions of living with chronic illnesses.

Rupp, Joyce. *Praying Our Good-Byes*. Notre Dame, IN: Ave Maria Press, 1988.

This loving, prayerful guide illustrates how to say good-bye in a variety of life situations.

Schnall, Maxine. What Doesn't Kill You Makes You Stronger: Turning Bad Breaks Into Blessings. Cambridge, MA: Perseus Publishing, 2002.

A good resource on making the best of tragedy.

Seniors' Digest. Seattle-King County Advisory Council on Aging and Disability Services; http://www.seniorsdigest.org.

This service publishes an online magazine for adults over age fifty-five, their families, and the network of volunteers and professionals who work with them.

Siebert, Al. The Resiliency Advantage: Master Change, Thrive Under Pressure, and Bounce Back From Setbacks. San Francisco: Berrett-Koehler, 2005.

Award-winning guide to becoming more resilient. A must-read for every adult.

Siebert, Al. *The Survivor Personality*. New York: Perigee, 1996.
This is the classic book on "bouncing back."

Staudacher, Carol. *Men and Grief*. Oakland, CA: New Harbinger Publications Inc., 1991.
Staudacher has written a guide for men surviving the death of a loved one.

Sutton Holder, Jennifer, and Jann Aldredge-Clanton. *Parting: A Handbook for Spiritual Care Near the End of Life*. Chapel Hill, NC: University of North Carolina Press, 2004.
A sensitive and helpful guide.

Take Care! Self Care for the Family Caregiver. A quarterly newsletter published by the National Family Caregivers Association.
For newsletter and membership information (available at no cost to family caregivers in the United States), contact the association at http://www.nfcacares.org/ *or 800-896-3650.*

Time to Decide: Information about Health-Care Decisions for Aging Adults and Their Families. Seattle: The Church Council of

Greater Seattle, Taskforce on Aging. This excellent brochure is available by calling 206-525-1213.

Today's Caregiver. A free online newsletter.

Caregivers can request the newsletter or purchase a subscription to the print magazine at http://www.caregiver.com/ *or by calling 800-829-2734.*

Wilber, Ken. Grace and Grit: Spirituality and Healing in the Life and Death of Treya Killam Wilber. Boston: Shambhala Publications, 2001.

Ken Wilber recounts this touching true story of love and tenderness about his wife, Treya, who died of cancer when they were newly married.

Zerah, Aaron. *As You Grieve.* Notre Dame, IN: Sorin Books, 2001.

The author gives comforting words to the grieving from faith traditions around the world.

About the Authors

Dr. John Gibson has more than thirty-five years of experience as a life coach and counsellor, focusing on adult development, aging, and families. A graduate of both Columbia University and the University of Michigan, he holds degrees in psychology, social work, applied statistics and a specialization in aging, focusing on adult development and family relationships. He has been on the faculty at Columbia University and the University of Washington. John coaches and speaks on topics related to multigenerational family relationships, wellness and illness, and building networks and community. He is the author of numerous articles and books on health, family, and aging. He has spoken internationally and has appeared on radio and television shows. John regularly consults with individuals and families, and frequently helps them set up personal safety nets or create care-share teams.

Judy Pigott has a wealth of extended, blended, and chosen family experiences in both leading and participating in care-share teams. She has an undergraduate degree in psychology from Skidmore College and a master's degree in teaching from Teachers College, Columbia University. Judy's post-graduate studies at Seattle University focused primarily on teaching English as an Additional Language. She also has training and experience in Hospice work and creating care-share teams. She is committed to fostering communities that nurture all participants physically, intellectually, emotionally, and spiritually.

Made in the USA
San Bernardino, CA
01 February 2018